TRANSPLANT

To Matt.
Enjoy!

TRANSPLANT

A CARDIAC SURGEON'S STORY OF IMMIGRATION & INNOVATION

Arvind Koshal

DR. ARVIND KOSHAL

Apr. 24

BARLOW BOOKS

Library and Archives Canada Cataloguing in Publication data available upon request.

978-1-998841-07-3 (hardcover)
978-1-998841-12-7 (ebook)

Printed in Canada

Publisher: Sarah Scott
Cover design: Melissa Jun Koshal
Interior design and layout: Ruth Dwight

For more information, visit **www.barlowbooks.com**

Barlow Book Publishing Inc.
96 Elm Avenue, Toronto, ON
M4W 1P2 Canada

Disclaimer

The events recounted in this memoir are based on the author's best recollections of personal experiences, conversations, and observations. While every effort has been made to ensure accuracy, the passage of time and the inherent fallibility of memory may result in slight variations from the precise details of certain events, dates, and conversations.

This memoir is a true reflection of the author's life as he remembers it, but it is important to acknowledge that personal perspectives and interpretations may differ among individuals who were present during these events. The author has striven to present an honest and sincere account of his experiences, but readers should keep in mind that memory is subjective and that the recollections contained herein are filtered through the author's perspective.

Additionally, the names and identifying details of certain individuals have been changed or omitted to protect their privacy. Any resemblance to real persons, living or deceased, is purely coincidental.

The purpose of this memoir is to offer readers a glimpse into the author's life and the lessons he has learned along the way. It is not intended to be a comprehensive historical or factual record, and readers are encouraged to approach its contents with an open and critical mind.

For my beloved wife, Arti

Contents

Foreword

by The Honourable Gary G. Mar, ECA, KC

President and CEO, Canada West Foundation

first met Dr. Arvind Koshal in 1999, when I had just been appointed Alberta's minister of health. We met for breakfast in my office, under the famous portrait Yosef Karsh had taken of a fuming Winston Churchill. Dr. Koshal came to the meeting with a very big ask: he wanted the government to fund a best-in-class centre for cardiac care. If agreed to, this would be a huge outlay of resources for the Government of Alberta, money both for capital costs to build it and, more significantly, for operating costs in perpetuity.

Dr. Koshal came to the meeting well prepared. He was well briefed on my background, and he had anticipated my questions and concerns. Even more important, he demonstrated the skills found in successful politicians: the ability to convey a story about why a cardiac centre would be important to Albertans. As he sipped his cup of tea, with milk and sugar, Dr. Koshal portrayed a vision for what a high-performance cardiac centre would mean for Alberta, and how we could mitigate the burden of cardiac disease. By the end of break-fast, he had convinced me. I wanted to share his vision. This was a vision that could make all Albertans proud.

The result was the Mazankowski Alberta Heart Institute, a remark-able achievement that has significantly reduced the waiting time for heart surgery. It was also an extraordinary achievement for Dr. Koshal, so when he asked me to write the Foreword to his memoir, I didn't hesitate to say yes. I wanted to gain further insight into the mind and background of a person who contributed so much to Alberta and to Canada.

This book is, in part, the memoir of an apprentice: the story of the transformation of a student of medicine to a practitioner of cardiac surgery. Other surgeons have written memoirs, such as Dr. William Nolan, who wrote *The Making of a Surgeon* in 1970. Both Nolan and Koshal write about the significance of mentors and teams, and the importance of treating patients with dignity and compassion. They both agree that patient outcomes are at the centre of medical decisions and that good communication is at the heart of good patient care.

Transplant, however, goes beyond the story of physician training. It is a story arc that covers three continents and innumerable cultures. It commences in India. From his birth, it was determined that Arvind would be a surgeon, like his father before him. And, like his father before him, his bride Arti was arranged for him. To Western culture, this may seem like a foreign concept indeed. Equally foreign to a Westerner might be the author's frequent references to the centuries-old Hindu scripture, the Bhagavad Gita. But to Arvind Koshal, these decisions and philosophy are deeply embraced and were an important part of his success and not a hindrance.

The Gita provided the author with guidance and the temperament to be a great doctor. Doctors are not gods. They are humans who should always endeavour to do their best. And they should be humble enough to acknowledge that a good patient outcome is the result of many people on a team. Doubtless, there are many grateful patients who will express gratitude to their surgeon for a successful outcome. But the Gita reminds its reader that "you are only entitled to the action, never its fruits."

The gold-medal student who had worked at a government-run medical college hospital in Raipur faced significant cultural differences when he came to train in Canada. The egalitarian treatment of patients in Ottawa was eye-opening. So too were the possibilities for the advancement of the field of cardiac care. In 1967, Dr. Christiaan Barnard had completed the first successful human heart transplant. Arvind Koshal wanted to make a difference in improving cardiac patient care, and there was a greater opportunity in Ottawa than in India. This led to the emotional decision to tell his family that he would remain in Canada to further his knowledge and not return to India. Punctuating the narrative of his training are vignettes of what it is like coming to a foreign land where helpful neighbours teach you how to remove snow from the driveway or warn you how not to light a gas barbecue. And where after long days of work you are comforted by Arti's preparation of a meal reminiscent of a home and family that are thousands of miles away.

Dr. Willie Keon is a significant character in this memoir. One can see the influence on Arvind Koshal when the author describes Dr. Keon: hard-working, superb surgeon; quiet, thoughtful, and skillful administrator. Dr. Koshal, too, is all of those things. Throughout his professional journey, the author evinces his capacity to learn, not only in the surgical suite but also in the boardroom. Whether it is a firm rebuke to an arrogant surgeon to treat a nurse with respect, the appropriate use of humour to disarm a contentious administrative logjam, or comforting words to a patient or family, Arvind learns from his own experience as well as that of others.

One may ask, can such a memoir also be a love story? The answer is yes. It is quite clear that Arti's love and support is with Arvind throughout his journey. The author acknowledges this in every aspect of his life and also credits her with the raising of three successful sons, Arjun, Anu, and Amit. Beyond support, Arti also provides guidance in Arvind's decisions, and this story is as much about her as it is about him.

You may not have met Arvind. You may not know what his profession was. But if you watched him cooking a meal, your Sherlockian powers of observation may cause you to conclude that he was a surgeon. His set-up, mise en place, is always the same. Carefully cut ingredients are laid out on the prep table. His culinary instruments are beside the cooking surface. The protein being cooked is tied with surgical knots. The pan is properly preheated to ensure the Maillard reaction between amino acids and sugars results in a delicious browning of the food. Instant-read temperature probes ensure that the dish, especially fish, is not overcooked.

There were great advancements in cardiac care over the course of this story. Heart disease is no longer the number one cause of death in Canada. Dr. Koshal's efforts contributed to that result. Many patients and families are grateful that Arvind's family chose for him to go to medical school and not the Cordon Bleu. He has achieved much, and deserves much credit, although he should still learn to tie his own shoes.

On April 7, 2010, Dr. Arvind Koshal was invested in the Order of Canada. His citation reads as follows:

> One of our leading cardiac surgeons, Arvind Koshal has significantly contributed to the advancement of health care in Canada. He has performed innovative techniques that have been adopted across the country, and was on the team that conducted the first total heart implant in Canada. He also performed the nation's first implantation of a left ventricular assist device, a small pump that improves blood flow. As the chief cardiac surgeon with the Capital Health Authority and the University of Alberta, he has developed its cardiac program into one of the largest in Canada. He has also been instrumental in the creation and development of the Mazankowski Heart Institute, one of the most advanced cardiac care centres in the country.

Introduction

My destiny was largely predetermined by my parents, who made two crucial choices in India that have shaped my path. The first, made before I was born, was that I would become a surgeon. The second, made after I finished medical school, was that I would marry Arti in an arranged marriage. Neither they, nor I, could have foreseen how far these decisions would take me.

Initially, I began writing these words to provide our children with a glimpse into their father's background. However, as the words flowed, I realized the magnitude of the story that needed to be shared. It is a tale that attests to opportunities given and risks taken, to what leadership and partnership can accomplish, to how and why heart disease is no longer the leading cause of death in Canada. That last bit is very good news for every Canadian as it resonates with our shared understanding of how profoundly heart-related issues can affect our lives and loved ones. It is a tale that transcends borders and sheds light on the imperfect yet remarkable progress of cardiac care in this extraordinary country.

This book is about how things unfolded from someone who lived and worked in the midst of that tale for over four decades.

It is also, in part, a response to the fact that most of us over the age of thirty-five have either personally sought or know a friend or family member who has sought cardiac advice. I've been on the surgeon side of those conversations thousands of times. I came to realize that many patients found comfort and assurance in the recommended procedure when they knew something of how we got to where we were and why we—and they—could trust the course of action to restore, or at least improve, their heart health. Framed around my personal journey, I wanted to offer readers a straightforward and accessible account of what has happened in heart surgery over the years to help us recognize the intricacies and appreciate the outcomes of what has occurred in the treatment of heart disease.

SINCE MY EARLIEST days as a doctor, I was driven by a desire to improve care for patients, irrespective of their means, and by the belief that there are ways to accomplish that through commitment and collaboration. After the first chapter, which describes my childhood, the rest of this book chronicles how this desire and belief came to both infuse and direct my life's work from India to Canada. I set the stage with some highlights in this introduction, but the chapters that follow provide the insider details that tell the fuller tale of how the landscape of cardiac care in Canada came to be transformed.

Fresh out of medical school in the early 1970s in India, I worked in a government-run hospital. Long waits, insufficient beds, and outdated equipment were the norm. Cardiac and thoracic surgery were almost nonexistent, leaving patients with little to no options when it came to life-saving procedures. This was a common reality during that era in many parts of India, where I was raised. I found those circumstances distressing and disheartening.

In 1975, newly married, I arrived at the Ottawa Civic Hospital for further training in general surgery. My wife, Arti, and I fully intended to return to India; however, my path took an unexpected turn. I made the decision to specialize in cardiac surgery, and we made the decision to establish our family in Canada. At that time, heart disease was the leading cause of death in Canada, claiming almost one-half of all deaths in the country.[1] Countless others experienced hospitalizations, disabilities, or a diminished quality of life due to the burden of heart disease. The field held immense potential for saving lives. Addressing this urgent need for improved access to advanced cardiac care was a circumstance I couldn't ignore.

Fortuitously, I found myself at the Ottawa Heart Institute at a time of significant growth in cardiac surgery. Under the guidance of Dr. Wilbert Keon, a prominent figure in cardiac care in Canada, our surgical team pioneered advanced procedures, techniques, and research. With new developments, more lives were saved, quality of care was improved, and patient mortality rates were reduced. All of this took place within Canada's health care system. It was truly remarkable to be a part of this groundbreaking era.

Fifteen years later, in 1991, I assumed the position of chief of cardio-vascular surgery at the University of Alberta Hospital in Edmonton. Cardiovascular disease still held its place as the primary cause of death in Canada. While the Canadian health care system provides quality care, access for non-urgent cases remained suboptimal. At that time, Alberta's waitlist for elective heart surgery stretched to over a year and a half, resulting in some patients deteriorating or even succumbing to their conditions. Challenges within the pediatric heart surgery program meant patients were transported to California for treatment. This was an untenable situation that demanded imme-diate action and reforms, which is what happened—though not as quickly as I and others would have hoped.

Over the following years, an incredible collaborative effort unfolded. Colleagues, administrators, political leaders, nurses, business figures, and countless others joined forces to revolutionize the delivery and quality of cardiac care in Alberta. The wait time for elective surgery was dramatically reduced to less than two weeks, the pediatric cardiac surgery program became one of the nation's best, and we solidified our position as the sole heart transplant centre serving Alberta, Saskatchewan, and Manitoba. And in 2008, the Mazankowski Alberta Heart Institute opened as one of North America's most advanced cardiac care centres for adults and children. It represented, for me, tangible evidence of what desire and belief could accomplish for patients and for Canada.

As you'll read, this transformative journey called on me to embrace multiple roles: perpetual learner and teacher, doctor, administrator, and someone who both offers and seeks help. This calling has filled each day of my life with profound meaning. Yet, as I reflected on the path travelled, I also realized the sacrifice it called for. Of sleep, time with my family, and, often, my own well-being—not unlike for many of my colleagues. There was also the sacrifice it called for from our families. That too is part of this tale.

A FEW YEARS ago, heart disease relinquished its status as the leading cause of death in Canada,[2] a remarkable milestone achieved through significant innovations in the medical field and increased awareness of preventive care. I am grateful to have been part of numerous exceptional teams that contributed to this progress. These contributions have not only saved countless lives but also improved the quality of life for patients across Canada, offering hope and brighter futures to those affected by heart disease.

1

Roots

My father's upbringing traces back to a humble village in Punjab, India. In that small corner of the world, my grandfather, a landlord, owned a handful of modest houses that he rented out to others. They lived in a spacious house with no electricity. Surrounding them were fields and cows, and the family sustained itself through farming wheat and rice. My grandmother dedicated her time to the kitchen and cooked delicious food. Education eluded my grandparents, yet they embraced the simplicity of their surroundings.

During scorching summer visits, our three generations would all congregate in a single room, seeking solace from the heat. A canvas sheet dangled from the ceiling, and a servant's deft manoeuvring of an attached rope created a makeshift fan, offering respite from the sweltering conditions. At night, we slept under the open sky, protected by mosquito nets, thankful for the cooler temperatures that prevailed after dusk.

A highlight of those annual visits was undoubtedly my grand-mother's cooking. She skillfully crafted parathas, a type of stuffed Indian bread, alongside dal, a lentil dish served with a generous dollop of butter and accompanied by the flatbreads known as roti. Although she spoke sparingly, her warm smile illuminated the room. These gatherings were filled with delightful conversations and infectious laughter. We went on walks to a nearby river, the very same waters where my father had spent his early childhood and learned to swim. There, with no formal lessons, he was dropped in, experiencing a true "sink-or-swim" lesson.

Despite my grandparents' lack of formal education, they placed great importance on ensuring my father received a proper education. He attended King Edward Medical College in Lahore, pursuing his ambition to become a surgeon. Thanks to my grandparents' savings, my father went to England to continue his studies, but not before fulfilling the prerequisite of marrying a suitable Indian girl.

The marriage was arranged with a young eighteen-year-old from the Sondhi family in Jalandhar. The Sondhis, a large family, boasted a higher education for most of their members. My mother, my father's bride-to-be, had attended college and obtained a bachelor of arts degree. Besides her academic achievements, she possessed remarkable skills in the kitchen, as well as in knitting and sewing. Soon after their wedding in 1946, they embarked on a momentous journey, which is difficult to fathom today. Thankfully, they did not endure the long and treacherous voyage around the Cape of Good Hope which many previous generations of Indians had braved to reach

England. Instead, they travelled through the Suez Canal, along the Gibraltar coast, passing one British colonial outpost after another, and eventually reaching the United Kingdom.

The aftermath of the Second World War loomed large in Europe, with extensive efforts underway to rebuild ravaged regions. England, having suffered significant bombing, was at the nascent stages of reconstruction. Bombed-out sites were scattered throughout the land-scape. Meanwhile, India yearned for the long-awaited independence promised to its people. Given Britain's own challenges on its home soil, the time seemed ripe for India to break free. Although it must have felt awkward for my father to move to the country that had dom-inated India for so long, England offered the best opportunities for advanced medical training. The boat journey was difficult, especially for my mother, who, pregnant with their first child, experienced a miscarriage either on board or shortly after their arrival—a poignant detail that was never made clear to me as a child.

LIVING IN POST-WAR England proved challenging. The linger-ing effects of the war were palpable, with most food still subject to rationing, inadequate heating in homes, and frequent blackouts plunging homes into darkness. Against this backdrop, my mother grappled with a profound sense of loneliness. She yearned for the familiar embrace of her family, not to mention the essential ingre-dients required to prepare a wholesome Indian meal. The absence of household help only intensified her plight. As I would later discover, she cried every day. While my father diligently pursued his studies as a full-time student, his commitments left him with limited avail-ability, further isolating my mother. Financially, they relied on the support provided by their parents, another difficult undertaking as our family expanded.

My sister, Reeni, came first, born in April 1947 at Hammersmith Hospital, a few months before India finally achieved independence. In May 1948, I came along. My name, Arvind, means "lotus," but my pet name was *Babbal*, with Reeni always calling me *Babli*. I can still hear her calling, "Babli, Babli!" To everyone else, however, I was, and am, Arvind.

I was born at the North Middlesex Hospital in the Registration district of Edmonton. Yes, Edmonton, a name that would later res-onate with the city in Alberta, Canada, where I would spend the greater part of my professional career. Was this a mere coincidence or a subtle harbinger of things to come? Being born in England, I was granted British citizenship, an advantage I called upon many years later to pass along to my three sons.

My father devoted countless hours to attending lectures and receiving private tutoring from esteemed British surgeons, all in preparation for the Fellowship examination of the Royal College of Surgeons. Among his mentors was the renowned professor of sur-gery at the Royal Postgraduate Medical School in Hammersmith, Ian Aird. Dr. Aird held distinction not only for his medical prowess but also for his voluminous textbook, *A Companion in Surgical Studies*, an impressive opus stretching to a weighty 999 pages.[3] Eschewing illustrations, Dr. Aird believed that diagrams oversimplified the subject matter. (Keep this in mind if you find yourself yearning for more diagrams in this more modest work of mine, which, thankfully, falls short of Aird's magnum opus in length!)

My father's big day came when he had to appear before the examiners at the Royal College. The final evaluation included both a written and an oral component. The written part assessed knowledge and the oral exam assessed clinical judgment. Before a surgeon would be allowed to operate, he had to obtain the FRCS—Fellowship of the Royal College of Surgeons—qualification.

At the oral examination, patients were strategically placed before the candidates, becoming subjects for their examination and subjects of questioning on diagnosis and treatment. Two examiners assessed every patient encounter, creating an atmosphere of unnerving scrutiny. As a candidate hailing from (newly liberated) India, my father undoubtedly confronted not only the intensity of the examination but also the shadow of deeper scrutiny, if not outright prejudice.

Shortly after the gruelling examination, candidates gathered in a room for the announcement of individual outcomes. Those who failed would seek solace in a bar downstairs, while the successful would be congratulated upstairs. Overwhelmed and anxious, my father initially said he wouldn't stay for the results or go to the podium, but my determined mother insisted on his presence. A close friend of my father, Dr. Sethi, had accompanied my mother. The dispute was settled when my father asked Dr. Sethi to go up to the podium in his place. Upon hearing that he had failed, Father planned to go down the stairs to the bar. Sethi was dubious about the plan but agreed after some persuasion. The ceremony began and when the master of ceremonies called "Krishan Dev Koshal," Sethi walked up and shook the chief examiner's hand.

"Congratulations, Dr. Koshal, you passed the examination," the man said.

A bewildered Sethi did not know what to do. He ran down the stairs shouting, "I am not Dr. Koshal!" He grabbed my father and said, "You passed, you idiot"—along with a few other choice words.

My father ran back up to the podium, but by then they had started calling the rest of the candidates. He sincerely wondered if his ruse would disqualify him permanently. He might never become a surgeon at all! He waited and waited. After a few other names were called, his was called again.

He went up to the podium where he was asked, "Are you sure you are Dr. Koshal?"

"I am and I am very sorry," he replied sheepishly.

The examiners congratulated him. Mother and Dr. Sethi joined him, all delighted with his achievement.

A few days later, Dr. Koshal, now adorned with the esteemed initials FRCS (London) after his name, embarked on the journey back to New Delhi, accompanied by his young family. No longer subjected to the arduous voyage by ship, they soared through the skies in a Douglas Dakota airplane—an emblem of human ingenuity forged in times of conflict, repurposed to carry civilians in peacetime across vast distances.

For me, a mere six months old, this momentous homecoming held little significance. Unaware of the damp, grey landscape of my birthplace, England, slowly fading from view, I was about to be immersed in the vibrant tapestry of my homeland, India. It was a land where the scent of fragrant spices and the ethereal aroma of burning incense filled the air, where sun-drenched days enveloped bustling streets teeming with life. Bells chimed, sirens blared, horns honked, voices melded into a symphony of sounds, harmonizing with the calls of birds and the ever-present rumble of traffic. This was the auditory mosaic that would shape my formative years, an indelible backdrop to the narrative of my childhood.

ONE OF MY earliest recollections transports me back to my days at a Montessori school, in Gwalior, where my parents were fervent advocates of my receiving a robust education in English. Their conviction stemmed from the belief that fluency in the language was essential if I were to become a doctor. After all, most medical textbooks were in English, not Hindi. Each day, a massive blue school bus would arrive to collect me, dwarfing our seemingly minuscule black Ford Prefect. The sight of it led my young mind to ponder on the significance of the driver's role—a person of great importance, surely.

My father, time and again, even in my tender years, would impress upon me the notion that I was destined to be a surgeon. "What do you aspire to be when you grow up?" he would inquire. "A surgeon," was my steadfast reply. But on occasion, a new idea would arise within me. "A bus driver," I declared once, provoking a flare of anger from my father. "Remember, you are meant to be a surgeon," he sternly reiterated. Determined to explore further, I ventured a new response on a subsequent occasion. "A sister," I mused, envisioning the kind nurses my father worked with—the term "sister" being synonymous with nurses in both India and England. Yet, the resounding refrain persisted: a surgeon, and nothing less.

My sister Reeni and I were very close, in age and in temperament. We never fought. Once we had some sort of disagreement and she wanted to get me in trouble. She scrawled on a wall in crayon, "This was written by Babli," as though I had done it. I don't remember that either of us got punished. But then again, there was no spanking at home, and it was rare to hear my parents ever raise their voices even with each other—unless they were fighting over a bridge game.

Born prematurely, I entered the world weighing less than five pounds. My parents, eager for me to thrive, encouraged me to consume greater quantities of nourishment. Milk, regarded as a complete food at the time, was deemed indispensable. It wasn't until later that information emerged highlighting its iron deficiency, emphasizing the need for a more balanced diet.

In India the milk was delivered directly to our house and was not pasteurized. To make it drinkable it had to be boiled. I hated hot milk, especially in the hot summer months. I much preferred the food at our school. It was served on stainless-steel plates with us seated cross-legged on the ground to eat it. My favourite dish was the curried potatoes with cilantro leaves. That and poori, a puffy deep-fried bread. Even now, at my age, I find immense pleasure in these simple yet flavourful dishes, often surpassing more extravagant fare.

It was a tradition in our family to have a "sweet dish" after dinner. They were mostly Indian dishes, such as rice or bread pudding and other milk-based desserts, plus the ubiquitous Jell-O. Caramel custard trifle and gateau mocha were reserved for special occasions with guests.

Despite their devotion to sweets, my parents harboured concerns about my weight and physical activity—or rather, the lack thereof, as I was far from athletic. Their remedy? Jumping jacks—a daily ritual that we partook in as a family. For years on end, even during my time in medical school, we faithfully engaged in this shared exercise, an enduring symbol of their commitment to my well-being.

The intricacies of India's class divisions can prove elusive to Westerners, yet they permeate the cultural fabric so profoundly that questioning them rarely arises during one's upbringing. Coming from a highly educated English-speaking family, we bore a distinctive marker. India boasts the second-largest English-speaking population globally, surpassed only by the United States. However, it is worth noting that merely a fraction of the nation possesses fluency in the language—a striking reminder of the country's staggering population density. English holds official status as one of India's twenty-two national languages, alongside Hindi. While travelling through the country, it is almost a certainty to encounter another English speaker, but nuances persist, ranging from our distinct accents to the multitude of words and phrases that have become uniquely our own.

In line with the prevailing customs of well-educated households, we employed two full-time maidservants. Kasturi bai served as our cook, while Sheila bai shouldered the responsibilities of cleaning, laundry, and, of course, attending to my needs. The honorific suffix "bai" conveys respect, and over the course of fifteen years or more, both became integral members of our family. Sheila bai, in particular, took charge of dressing me and preparing me for school. Even after I had completed high school, she insisted on tying my shoelaces—an endearing routine that endured. Each year, as a gesture of appreciation, we presented them with new saris on their birthdays. While not the most extravagant garments, they had to be respectable enough to flaunt proudly among our neighbourhood's other maidservants.

After Montessori school I went to the prestigious Scindia School in Gwalior where we lived. Originally meant for sons of Indian royalty and nobility, it was high on a hill, built on top of an ancient historic fort. A "public" school—what would be termed a "private" school in North America—it was a boarding school almost by necessity. No caravan of school buses could have ever made it up and down that steep hill. When I was eight, my father was promoted to professor and head of the Department of Surgery in Jabalpur, several hours away by car. It was the middle of term, a bad time to change schools. I had to stay behind in Scindia at the posh boarding school.

What a tearful farewell that was, all of us crying. We were all devastated. I wouldn't be able to see my parents regularly, as I had in Gwalior. I would be able to join them at the end of term, but for now I was stuck. I had always had a good sense of humour and now it became a great source of comfort. I loved to tell jokes, and at Scindia I now had a new and appreciative audience. Even in that brief time

I was voted the best comedian among my group of boys at Scindia, a point of honour.

In Jabalpur our first house was a rental of about 1,800 square feet, a little smaller than our previous home. There was a master bedroom for my parents, a small office for my father, small bedrooms for Reeni and me, a dining room, one bathroom for all of us, and, at the back of the house, quarters for our three maidservants. Almost every room had ceiling fans plus air conditioning units we'd put in the windows come summer, not to mention portable swamp coolers. Best of all, it was close to my new school—Christ Church Boys' High School. I could walk or ride my bike there, and one of the maids could bring me a hot lunch in a tiffin carrier, food I often shared with a friend who didn't have such a luxury. I had to wear a white shirt, khaki pants, a green blazer with yellow stripes, and a green-and-yellow tie. That sort of formality didn't seem unusual to me. After all, Father always wore a coat and tie.

Father also loved to garden. In the house we eventually built, he made sure there was a beautiful rose garden—with all sorts of colours—that he cared for plus a variety of red, white, green, yellow, and purple dahlias. He would even name the roses in the garden after members of the family. I could go outside and point to an Arvind rose and a Reeni rose. My father might have had a stiff upper lip, a remnant of his British training, but he was soft and warm on the inside. Never for a minute did I doubt his love.

Christ Church was a Protestant missionary school where once again all the teaching was in English. Hindi and Sanskrit were side

subjects—Sanskrit with its ancient roots would be a little like studying Latin or Greek in the West—but reading and writing in English
were crucial. My parents chose St. Joseph's Convent School for my
sister Reeni for similar reasons. It didn't have anything to do with reli-
gion—we were Hindu, after all. It was to make sure she had a solid
grounding in English. We could and did speak Hindi at home, mostly
with Kasturi bai and Sheila bai, but most often the family used English.

In Jabalpur, I stumbled upon a book—a book of jokes. Simple and
unadorned, it held no pretense of high literature or complex nar-
ratives. Just jokes. A compilation from the 1920s, deemed the best
by some English professor of yore. I spent the summer months
engrossed in its pages, committing joke after joke to memory, finding solace in the simple pleasure of laughter. Through the trials of
medical school and the demanding life of a doctor, that book became
my respite—a momentary escape from the weight of the world. And
later, as an immigrant in unfamiliar territory, it served as common
ground, a way to connect with others through shared humour.
Laughter, in its purest form, is a universal language that transcends
borders and brings people together. It breaks down barriers and eases
the tensions that separate us. In those moments of shared laughter, the world feels a little lighter, a little more bearable. That book
of jokes remains a cherished treasure—a reminder of the power of
laughter to uplift, to unite, and to remind us of our shared humanity.
And so, I turn to it time and again, finding solace and strength in the
simple act of laughter.

IN MANY WAYS our family straddled two cultures. My father and I dressed in coats and ties while my mother had a real taste for beautiful silk saris. In most Indian homes you would see a small altar with a statue of the deity they worshipped. We followed Arya Samaj, a monotheistic tradition, and therefore only had a simple statue. The biggest Hindu celebration comes in the fall, Diwali, the Festival of Lights, a little bit like Christmas in the West. There'd be fireworks, special scented candles, and lamps, but most significantly for me, sweets, lots of sweets—cashew fudge, white syrupy dumplings, sweet creamy noodles, sweet yogurt, nurturing a sweet tooth in me that hasn't left (true confession from a health-conscious cardiac surgeon!). We didn't go to a temple—worship was something to be done at home. We'd sit on a carpet on the floor and say our prayers together.

At Christ Church, one of the climaxes of the school year came with the annual elocution contest. The principal, Reverend Canon J.E. Robinson, was keen that I learn and recite "The Cataract of Lodore" by Robert Southey, English poet laureate from 1813 until his death in 1843. The poem was written in 1820 and describes the Lodore Falls at Keswick, formed by a small river from Watendlath Tarn that sends water tumbling across a hundred feet of enormous boulders, with a drop at one point of almost ninety feet.

"'How does the water / Come down at Lodore?' / My little boy asked me / Thus once on a time; / And moreover he tasked me / To tell him in rhyme." Other family members took up the request. "And 'twas in my vocation / For their recreation / That so I should sing; / because I was Laureate / To them and the King." Stanza after stanza filled my head: "From its sources which well / In the tarn on the fell; / From its fountains / Its rills and its gills…"

I learned it all by memory: "Helter-skelter / Hurry-skurry" so I could recite it dramatically by heart. How well did it stick? Even now, if you give me an hour I can still come up with the words, all the way to the end—a reverberating torrent of verbs: "And rushing and flushing and brushing and gushing, / And flapping and rapping and clapping and slapping, / And curling and whirling and purling and twirling … And so never ending, but always descending, / Sounds and motions for ever and ever are blending / All at once and all o'er, with a mighty uproar, / And this way the water comes down at Lodore."

I did so well with it that I won the contest that year, to the considerable pride of my beloved parents. First place! I don't remember what I recited the next year. Whatever it was, I was good enough to come in second. Not bad. And yet, when I came home and told my parents the good news, I could see the disappointment in Mother's eyes. Second place was okay, but not great. Especially if I was going to become a surgeon.

At age fifteen, I graduated from Christ Church and spent the next year preparing for the medical school entrance examination. Only about one in a hundred candidates ever passed. The pressure was on. I studied and studied. Perhaps the gift of memorizing an old poem had the added benefit of helping me learn by rote so many facts I would have to retain. Whatever it was, I passed. No disappointment in my parents' eyes this time. Just pride. I was on my way.

2

A Noble
Profession

I started my medical studies at the Government Medical College in Jabalpur, where we lived. It was only a bus ride away. Here the other students weren't just boys, as in high school, but also a lot of women. Even then, in 1965, fifty per cent of the medical students were women, who dressed in traditional saris and kurta. Very few in Western dress back then. They tended to be at the top of our class when it came to exam time, better prepared and more focused than us boys. As attractive as they were, we were all working so hard—or I was so shy—that there was no time for much flirtation. We were intent on becoming good doctors. Competition was intense and there was no room for failure or even second-best. I worked hard all day and studied all night, setting a pattern that would continue for years.

Anatomy and physiology were the principal subjects in the first two years. One of our first assignments was dissecting human cadavers. Picture it: a hundred students in a large room; all bent over some twenty cadavers; each, one at a time, putting our hands in to isolate a muscle or organ. For reasons that remain a mystery to me even to this day, we were not allowed to use gloves. Just our bare hands. After a day in the lab, we reeked of the formalin used for embalming. For weeks on end, I would come home stinking of a cadaver. No amount of handwashing could rid me of it. Indian food is eaten with the fingers, and as I dipped my fingers into a bowl and reached for my mouth, all I could smell was the formalin, not the delicious food. Mealtime, once a great joy, was no longer a pleasant experience.

Each of us was required to have a skeleton of our own. There were brokers—some a bit unsavoury—who would sell such things. If your skeleton was missing a certain bone, they'd assure you they could find it—for a price. You never wanted to know exactly where or how. I had a small scholarship, which was an extraordinary honour. To me, the honour itself was more important than the money. Naturally, it added to the pressure. I had to make sure I did well enough to qualify for the scholarship the next year, and the next.

For physiology, I had the privilege of being taught by Professor Mathur, whose profound impact on me extended far beyond his expertise. Interestingly, he had pursued his studies in Toronto—who could have foreseen that I would find myself studying in Canada just a few years later? Professor Mathur often reminded us of his connection to the very place where Banting and Best made the groundbreaking discovery of insulin in July 1921, subsequently earning them the esteemed Nobel Prize in medicine.

HOWEVER, FOR ME, Professor Mathur's most profound influence was in introducing me to the Bhagavad Gita, an ancient Hindu book of philosophy composed nearly three thousand years ago. In contrast to a religious sermon, it serves as a guiding light to comprehend life and navigate its intricacies. Through verses such as the following, its wisdom becomes apparent: "Anger gives rise to delusion. Delusion clouds one's memory and understanding, leading to the erosion of discernment. With the loss of discernment, a person's very existence is jeopardized."

Professor Mathur's insistence on exploring the profound insights contained within this ancient text opened my mind to a deeper understanding of existence and how to approach it.

That a professor of physiology would introduce me to such wisdom rocked me to the core. Being a good doctor was not just learning about parts of the body and how they function but also understanding the spirit within. Not just the heart but the soul. The art of the practice.

"He who holds his inner spirit unbound, whatever he may do, whose self is well controlled and who is free from desire, attains by such renunciation that supreme goal which is the aim of renunciation of action" is another passage. I began then the practice of reading a page of the Gita at the end of every day before going to bed, a practice I continue to this day. Things that I only half-understood then, in my late teens, have acquired greater meaning with the years. Here I was, constantly striving to do my best because nothing but the best was expected of me. How wonderful to have the Gita there to remind me not to measure my worth by achievement only. Not to look just for the reward.

"That gift is classed as pure which is made to one who is not expected to do something in return," says the Gita, "and is made with the feeling that the gift is a duty and is also made in the right place and time to a worthy person." Or this: "The same in honour and calumny, the same to friend and foe, having abandoned all worldly undertaking—such a one is declared as having overcome natural propensities." To meditate on such profound thoughts has given me and many others solace and comfort in countless difficult situations. It gives me perspective.

Throughout the years, I have immersed myself in diverse translations and interpretations of the Gita. However, my steadfast ritual remained unchanged: reading a page at the close of each day. There was one instance that stands out vividly in my memory. During a trip to Saudi Arabia, where the sight of carrying a non-Islamic text could potentially pose risks, I took extra precautions. I diligently photocopied a few pages of the Gita, ensuring their presence by my side. The significance of having those pages with me cannot be overstated. It held a profound meaning that resonated deeply within.

DURING MY TIME in medical school, years three to five were dedicated to the study of various clinical subjects, including surgery, medicine, ophthalmology, obstetrics, and gynecology. With our family's relocation from Jabalpur to Raipur, I transitioned to the Medical College at Ravishankar University. It's worth noting that the university shared a name that might ring familiar to many in the West, due to renowned sitarist and composer Ravi Shankar, although it was not named after him. It was at this institution that we experienced our initial interactions with patients.

Having grown up as the son of a surgeon, I had already witnessed the profound impact my father had on his patients. The simplest of procedures, like an appendectomy, could potentially save a life, leaving the recipients forever grateful. Even though my father occasionally exhibited arrogance and aloofness, stemming from his British medical training, the appreciation bestowed upon him by his patients was evident.

Now, here I was, witnessing with my own eyes the profound capacity of a doctor to alleviate human suffering—an ability that held the potential for me to do the same. As I have often expressed, the initial decision to embark upon the path of becoming a surgeon was not entirely mine. Yet, at this moment in my studies, I fully embraced it as my own. While some individuals might grapple with life choices seemingly dictated by their parents, I did not encounter such struggles. Deep within, I carried an unshakeable certainty that I was embarking upon a noble and remarkable profession.

THE INTERNSHIP THAT followed was a bit of a wake-up call. Visiting a primary care health centre in a nearby village gave me a perspective on the country's vast underfunding for medical care. The facilities were meagre and rundown. Often the first contact a patient had with a physician came in late stages of a disease such as tuberculosis and cancer. Patients were triaged to the nearby government city hospitals, but few followed the advice for fear of going to a big town or city, far from loved ones.

Dealing with patients with advanced disease was very disturbing. Women came in, often being seen for the first time, with advanced cases of breast cancers, occasionally with fungating (or ulcerating) masses.

We saw the results of heavy tobacco use and people smoking bidi, an unprocessed form of tobacco, highly addictive with three to five times more nicotine than a typical cigarette. It causes respiratory illness, oral cancer, and an inflammatory disease of peripheral blood vessels called Buerger's disease. The blood vessels narrow, which can prevent blood flow and cause clots to form. Patients would show up in severe pain with gangrene of feet and hands that required amputation. Those with no gangrene still had difficulty with pain control. And yet, even with unrelenting pain, the addiction to tobacco was so strong that they could not give up bidi. We'd see patients with amputated feet or hands still smoking. These encounters provided a painful yet invaluable lesson in the formidable grip of addiction, reinforcing the dire consequences that ensue when such forces gain dominion over individuals' lives.

We saw several cases of tuberculosis, affecting lungs, lymph nodes, intestines, and bones. The advent of anti-tubercular drugs had improved the results from previous years, but back then, in the late 1960s and early '70s, it was still present, often with debilitating results. I never saw a single case of tuberculosis after I arrived in North America.

Reports of unethical practices in small towns and villages were rampant. It was not unusual for a person not to have a last name and date of birth and have it replaced by an approximate age, usually incorrect. Uneducated, unaware, most of them lived day to day and had many children. Needless to say, they and their circumstances were easily exploited by unscrupulous doctors, some of whom had no medical qualifications whatsoever. I learned about a so-called doctor who had a small refrigerator filled with past patients' X-rays. He would claim to take X-rays by bringing the patient in front of the refrigerator, opening the door, and shutting it after the light was seen. If seeing someone with a possible arm injury, he would take out an old X-ray of somebody with a broken arm and show it to the patient. He then placed on a cast and charged the patient for the X-ray and cast.

There were other similar cases. A general practitioner had a very busy following with poor people. He was reputed to give an injection for well-being. As the story goes, on one occasion he mistakenly gave the injection to the patient's husband. When the man told him it was for his wife, the doctor told her to hold his hand for twenty minutes. As though that would do the trick.

At my graduation, there were no pass/fail stairways leading up and down as there had been for my father in England. What I do remember is going up to receive my first gold medal, for surgery. What an honour. I figured that would be it—good enough—but just as I was ready to head back to my seat, someone said, "You'd better stick around. There's more coming." And there were: for medicine, ophthalmology, obstetrics, and gynecology. Five gold medals in total. Plus, a few weeks after convocation: the Pfizer scroll of honour and gold medal for being an outstanding medical graduate. You can imagine how proud my parents were. The pride and joy radiating from my parents' faces surpassed any previous moment, even eclipsing the elation they had exhibited during my victory in the elocution contest. With the completion of my studies, I had earned the esteemed title of MBBS, signifying my attainment of a bachelor of medicine and surgery.

AFTER GRADUATION, I worked in the government-run Medical College Hospital in Raipur. What another eye-opening experience that was. Long lineups in the outpatient clinics and lack of hospital beds were the norm. The addition of "floor beds" was not uncommon, sometimes just a pillow and a mattress on the floor between beds. Nursing care was limited in quality and quantity. Nurses were not paid well and were treated harshly by the physicians, earning little respect. No wonder my father frowned at my notion of becoming a sister all those years ago. Now that I was a surgeon, I was seeing up close the downside of the profession in my country. Even in that government-run hospital, few medical records or patient charts were maintained and those that existed contained minimal information. Results of laboratory tests were not reliable.

The operating theatres had equipment dating back a few decades. There was no electrocautery to apply heat to tissue to control bleeding. Instead, you'd have to suture a bleeder by hand, which takes longer and is not as efficient. When it came to anesthesia, ether—considered obsolete even then—was still used. Because of toxicity and bad side effects, it was very much out of date.

Moreover, there were no ventilators for post-operative respiratory care. Once the surgery was concluded, the anesthesiologist would remove the endotracheal tube that had been inserted in the trachea, and if the patient could not breathe, they were left to die. There weren't any intensive care facilities.

During those years, disciplines like cardiac or thoracic surgery were non-existent, and esophageal surgery was only sporadically performed. General surgeons shouldered the responsibility of handling head injuries and other traumatic cases. Their expertise encompassed abdominal surgery, urological procedures, select head and neck surgeries, and rudimentary orthopedic care. Outpatient facilities were sparse, even for minor procedures. In addressing the prevalent issue of draining superficial abscesses, which accounted for approximately twenty patients per day, only two scalpel blades were available. After using one blade, it was swiftly replaced with the other one that had been immersed in an antiseptic solution after use on the previous patient. It was an era reminiscent of the Dark Ages. I acknowledge that considerable advancements have been made since then, but this was the early 1970s, a time marked by substantial gaps in medical infrastructure and resources.

Most patients who required intravenous glucose or saline infusions had to purchase them from outside the hospital. As junior doctors, we would keep any stock left over from other patients to use for very poor patients.

Wound infections were common even after simple procedures, a result of operating rooms that were not well sterilized. I could feel a tension building within me. The desire to heal and offer the best medical care possible—to be the surgeon I felt called to be—against overwhelming odds. I could see that same tension in my country. The poor government health facilities led to small private clinics with fee-for-service care. Some had a single operating room and six to ten patient rooms. These were cleaner and better maintained. Those who could afford it would use these facilities. But statistics of morbidity and mortality were not maintained anywhere.

The situation was different in the big cities where some of the government-run hospitals were much better equipped and maintained. For instance, the All India Institute of Medical Sciences (AIIMS) in New Delhi was a public facility that catered to VIPs and politicians from around the country (as I was to discover first-hand). The quality of medical and surgical staff was vastly superior. Most of the senior doctors had advanced training in the United Kingdom or North America and had brought their expertise home. And yet, there again lay that tension between personal goals and public service, when you learned that almost ninety per cent of the doctors who graduated from AIIMS went abroad. Most did not return home—a significant brain drain on the country.

In the cities, public facilities were crowded and difficult to access, with long waiting times. This led to small private facilities focused on individual specialties, such as obstetrics, general surgery, cataract surgery, and simple orthopedic operations. These were lucrative propositions for doctors and entrepreneurs, catering to those that could afford to pay. None of these options appealed to me.

As it had been determined by my parents (before I was born) that I would be a surgeon, I found myself taking up a position—in good part, thanks to my father—as house surgeon at the Medical College Hospital in Raipur. It offered me a wide range of opportunities to perform minor procedures and assist in major cases. At the same time, like my father, I knew I needed to pursue options to continue my study abroad—in my case North America, not England.

To be able to do that, I needed to take the Education Council of Foreign Medical Graduates (ECFMG) examination, a requirement for foreign medical graduates who wished to go to Canada or the United States. The examination had been banned in India to limit the brain drain of doctors. The nearest place to take it was in Ceylon, now Sri Lanka. I registered to take the exam in Colombo, the capital city. With its rich Buddhist history and culture, Sri Lanka was a popular destination for pilgrims. To get into the country, it was easiest to apply for a pilgrim's visa, as I did. On my return home, *The Times of India* had a front-page article with the heading: "Pilgrims Going to North America as Doctors." After that Sri Lanka did not allow doctors to come in as pilgrims.

I PASSED THE ECFMG examination, but before going abroad, my father suggested that I should go to New Delhi for more training and obtain a master of surgery at AIIMS. Once again, I faced fierce competition. Applicants came from across the country. In general surgery, they took only three or four candidates.

I was thrilled as were Mother and Father when I got in, but there would be another parting of ways. Other than a short time when I was eight, I had always lived at home with my parents and my sister, not to mention Sheila bai and Kasturi bai.

To get to New Delhi meant driving to the airport in Nagpur—there wasn't a good airport in Raipur yet, just a runway and single building—and then taking a two-hour flight to New Delhi. I had a tiny room at the student hostel, where I always had a kerosene lamp at hand to keep up my studies late at night, in case there was a blackout—which happened often enough. Our food was brought to us. There was no shower, and to heat water for a bath, we put these electrodes in the cold water to warm it up—not a very safe practice when I think about it. In the summer, if it got too hot, I could take my portable couch up to the roof and sleep there beneath the moon and stars.

Even amidst my intensive medical training, the family continued to take vacations together in the sweltering summer months, seeking the cooler mountain air. On the train, where there was no air conditioning, you could buy a huge block of ice and watch it melt through the journey as you hoped it cooled you off. We'd stay at places like the old Savoy Hotel in Mussoorie, overlooking the Garhwal mountain range, its classic English neo-Gothic architecture, a remnant of the British Raj. Back in the day it had been a refuge for the European overlords—at least now families like ours got to use it. We went to other hill stations, too, like Gulmarg at the base of the Himalayas (my first experience seeing snow on the ground). I loved going on long walks, breathing in the fresh air, savouring the blooming rhododendrons crowning the hills. Soon enough I'd be back at my books and the hospital, and the frantic urban world.

The professor of surgery at the AIIMS was Dr. Atm Prakash, a well-known and highly capable general surgeon. He had a great reputation and was well connected at the highest level of the federal government. How fortunate I was that he took me under his wing. It made all the difference. He was an excellent teacher. Even on weekends he would do teaching rounds for a few hours. We accompanied him in silent awe.

Most of the senior staff had trained abroad, and the academic sessions were of a high standard. After all, this was the best in India. And yet, there was not a lot of hands-on experience, so essential to becoming a surgeon. As a trainee, I would assist the assistant, who was usually the assistant professor. Of course, I learned a lot by watching, but not until I moved to Canada did I get that ongoing, regular scalpel-in-my-hands experience.

AIIMS attracted important government officials and politicians as patients. Across the street was the Safdarjung Hospital, a public facility, which was the trauma centre and handled most emergency patients. As such, we saw mainly non-emergency surgical cases. Among the VIPs we treated were Sanjay Gandhi, the son of Indira Gandhi, the prime minister, and Atal Bihari Vajpayee, who became prime minister a few years later. Here again, I witnessed the contrast between how the privileged were treated as opposed to the regular patients.

For instance—such a painful memory—we would have to treat outpatients who'd come in with swollen abscesses that needed to be drained. We'd operate on them with the most minimal anesthesia imaginable, at most a local spray. Not surprisingly they'd scream out in pain. You'd do your best to block out the sound as you did the necessary work.

I encountered a striking contrast when a VIP such as Sanjay Gandhi underwent a hernia operation. In this case, I received specific instructions to remain by his side in his room for a period of five days, attending to his needs during the recovery process. I questioned whether such disparities in treatment were unique to India or if I would encounter similar discrepancies elsewhere. Did the system inherently perpetuate caste and class differences? These experiences began to sow the seeds of my deep longing for a health care system that would offer universal and equitable treatment for all, irrespective of social standing. It was a yearning that fuelled my determination to fight for change.

One of the requirements for training was a research thesis. With the recommendation of Dr. Prakash, I wanted to use an old machine in the department to do internal gastric freezing for peptic ulcer treatment. This entailed introducing a balloon into a patient's stomach and running a cold solution into the balloon to temporarily freeze the stomach lining and the nerve endings. My hope was it would relieve the symptoms.

Peptic ulcer was a common enough ailment, and I had no difficulty recruiting patients for the study, done on an outpatient basis. Alas, my study showed no benefit of this modality. Still, I was grateful to be given the opportunity to pursue the idea and test it, something I'd have even greater experience with in Canada.

I had both a written exam and oral exam for master of surgery at AIIMS and passed them both, as well as being awarded the gold medal. My thesis was presented, and it was accepted. Dr. Prakash suggested that I apply to Canadian centres for further training in general surgery. He had trained in Canada and thought that would be a worthwhile endeavour for me. I wrote to several Canadian institutions and was accepted at the University of Ottawa. Because of the reputation of Dr. Prakash and AIIMS, I was admitted into general surgery as a third-year resident, a position not generally offered to a foreign medical graduate.

But before I could go—like my father before me—I needed to have a nice Indian wife.

3

The Right Match

Almost all marriages in India are arranged by the parents. They feel they know best what is right for their children. When a girl in India gets married, she not only marries the boy but also becomes part of his family. The premise of arranged marriages is to match socio-economic similarities of both partners. Parents feel that they can make decisions based on rational versus emotional values. They want to ensure financial security for their daughter. Love marriages certainly happened—as they did in my future bride's family—but they were uncommon.

Living in the West for so many years, I have often been asked how an educated person—like me—would agree to a system of arranged marriage. I can only speak from experience. After all, growing up in India, I had no other expectations or choice. It was what was done. At the time, I knew I didn't want to marry another physician, or anybody associated with the health profession for that matter. Those were the people I had to work with and interact with every day. I hoped for something different. How would I find that on my own? I hardly had the time. Then again, I knew my parents would be discerning in selecting my bride and I did not want to disappoint them. Per usual.

Most dating when I was growing up in India felt very superficial. I remember having a female friend in New Delhi whom I liked very much. We got together a few times but when I realized that my parents would be looking for a bride for me very soon, I discontinued the relationship. I didn't want to give her the wrong impression. I felt bad about it, but I think it was the right decision. I didn't want to lead her on. While I was training in general surgery, my parents had been talking for over a year with a family that was of a similar caste and social status as our own, Punjabis by background like us. The arrangement was made largely through our friends Mrs. Arjun Singh and her daughter Veena, who happened to be the roommate of my bride-to-be. Mr. Arjun Singh himself was a prominent politician in India who served in multiple state and national roles—obviously a vote of confidence for us—and although I didn't know it, his daughter Veena had had her eye on me as a perfect match for Arti for some time. Two years earlier she had arranged for us to be together so that Arti could at least get a glimpse of me, across a not-too-crowded room. Seen from a distance, Arti was not entranced, not at all.

I'm short, five-foot-five, and have never weighed more than 140 pounds. I was even skinnier then. Arti took one glance and decided I looked like an eighth grader. A scrawny kid, not the classic dreamboat of tall and handsome. No way was she interested. Veena did not give up though. She knew enough about me and our families through years of friendship and association. In fact, my father had saved her mother's life years earlier, flying across the country and operating on her for peritonitis. Knowing a surgeon wasn't such a bad thing. Give it a few years. Arti and her family would surely come around.

When matchmaking resumed in earnest, the two families took a closer look at each other. Arti's family seemed very similar to mine: middle-class, well-educated professionals. Her father was a mining engineer and had served in the government. At the time he was on a UN assignment in Lesotho in Southern Africa. Arti herself had graduated from college with a degree in home economics and education, and had recently begun teaching in Lesotho.

Yet with all those apparent similarities, the families were different in other ways. Her father was well-travelled, having spent several months in the United States as a young man. When Arti, the first-born, was only three years old, he arranged for an aunt and uncle to care for her while he and her mother went off to Europe for three months, to see the world. He wanted his four daughters to be women of the world, too, not just dutiful housewives. Arti would say of her upbringing, "we were raised to think about what the world had to offer." Very different from the expectations of a typical, well-raised "nice" Indian girl who was expected to focus on the family and the home. Even as a home economics major—as I was to discover—Arti had very little kitchen experience. She wasn't expected to simply become a good cook.

From far-off Southern Africa, Arti's father wrote letters to his contacts to find out all he could about my family. Due diligence. Anything they should know about us. Trying to get it right. At least there wasn't any expectation of lavish gifts, money, or jewellery from us. Just the right match. It all looked very promising.

With Arti in distant Lesotho, photos had to be exchanged. I was asked to go to one of the photographers in Connaught Place in New Delhi to have my picture taken. "Are you married or are you happy?" the photographer asked—a joke I didn't quite get. Or was it one? He then asked if this photo shoot was for a marriage proposal. Yes, I said. I hadn't grown any taller but by now I had a moustache and apparently looked more suitable. Not an eighth grader.

Still, as Arti would tell you, it surprised her that she accepted the arrangements without any second thoughts. Her younger sisters, in fact, went on to be those rare cases in India of love matches, not arranged marriages. It says a lot about her family. "I was used to speaking out for myself, sharing my opinion," Arti says. "I went to a girls' private high school, after all." And yet, she found herself mostly listening when it came to this marriage possibility. "I thought of myself as a modern woman. And here I was, going for something that felt like a toss of the coin." She had to trust what her parents thought. No decision would be made quickly. And she could change her mind at any time. One of the things she never would have abided was living as a joint family as is usually the case in India—multiple generations in one household. Who could have guessed that would never be the case with us? Talk about a coin toss!

The detective work on both sides continued. My parents were still in Raipur, and they were quite satisfied with the credentials of Arti's family because of the various connections we had through friends. Not to mention the common friendship of matchmaking Veena.

I got a message from home that I was to come to Raipur to meet a prospective bride. A couple of days before I was leaving, Veena's mother called me, which was unusual: she suggested very clearly that I should like her choice. The fix was in.

I flew to Raipur. At the same time Arti's family arrived from Southern Africa via Bombay and was staying at another friend's house. Traditionally, the two families initially meet without the prospective bride present. This is in case something does not work out that would expose the girl to the other family and cause disappointment. I later learned that prior to this visit, Arti's family had seen nine other boys and had turned them down. Incalculable odds.

When the family arrived for lunch at our house, I sat next to the prospective father-in-law. I showed him my letters of reference for Canada. My parents talked about the fact that I had been on the team that had operated on Indira Gandhi's son, little realizing that Arti's parents were not fans of the prime minister.

The following day was the first time I saw Arti. She looked beautiful in her sari, about my height which was a bit of a relief—at least she wouldn't tower over me. But we were kept far apart and didn't have any conversation together. After they left, I didn't say anything to my parents—not that I was expected to. They were doing all the heavy lifting. And I completely trusted their judgment.

The two families met again the next day at our home (not that we could have gathered in Arti's home all the way in Africa). In the presence of both sides, my mother asked me if I was agreeable to go ahead with marrying Arti. I responded yes, without any hesitation. Essentially, we got engaged without talking to each other. That it worked out so beautifully is beyond comprehension. With each year we've grown closer, more grateful for each other. I could not have done what I've done without Arti, and she couldn't possibly have known what huge demands my career would make on her. But there we were, two young people whose lives would be inextricably bound.

We met briefly at lunch. I told her the only way this would work out was if both of us were adaptable. In this arrangement, we love the person we marry.

"I have never grown up with a lot of wealth so I'm quite comfortable being adaptable," she said. She had no idea what a surgeon's life was like. She asked me what kind of a surgeon I was.

I replied, "a general surgeon."

"So, what does a general surgeon do?" she asked.

"We perform gallbladder, hernia, and other abdominal surgery," I said.

"Why could you not be a brain surgeon or heart surgeon?"

"Those specialties are labour- and time-intensive. I would not get married if I was to succeed in either of those specialties." Famous last words.

One conversation I never heard was what her mother said about me. "That he's well educated and has done well professionally is what counts. So what if he's a little short? You can't have everything."

Two weeks later we got married—hardly a long engagement. My professor, Atm Prakash, had warned me not to get married during my residency. He felt that once residents got married, they didn't work hard. He was a bit disappointed but got over it. I had two days off from work, and if we took advantage of the weekend, we'd find the necessary time.

Indian weddings go on for at least three days: one day of singing; one for the formal engagement; and a day for the ceremony, which can be long and tedious. The latter took place at the Oberoi Intercontinental Hotel in New Delhi on November 25, 1974. Because of a national famine at the time and government restrictions, we could only have one hundred guests—a big contrast to what was normal, with hundreds of guests welcome. We did our best to extend the guest list, holding a larger reception at another venue the next day. In attendance were all my surgical colleagues, some of my teachers, and such luminaries as my former patient Sanjay Gandhi, the politician Atal Bihari Vajpayee who later became the prime minister of India, and, of course, Arjun Singh with his wife and their daughter Veena, beaming with pleasure and so instrumental in bringing Arti and me together.

As is traditional, for the ceremony, I got on a white horse at my aunt and uncle's house to ride to the hotel, with friends and family gathered around, hailing the bridegroom. But as this was teeming New Delhi, even at one-seventh of the population it has today, I couldn't ride all the way to the Oberoi Intercontinental. Too many cars, too many people. I got off, the horse went on ahead, we all got in cars, and then at the entrance to the hotel, I got out of the car and back on the horse. There was a live band with bugles, trumpets, and people dancing around me. Arti was late, as usual—good to get used to that—but then, there she was: my beautiful bride.

We flew to Raipur for the second reception with my family and our friends, with multiple invitations to our close friends' homes, as is customary. There was plenty of good food and lots of dancing, but truth be told, I'm not much of a dancer. As agile as I could be with surgical instruments in my hands, I'm awkward on my feet. Arti, on the other hand, loves to dance and she looked great. At the end of the joyous celebrations, we returned to New Delhi, the newlyweds finally getting a chance to know each other. An arranged marriage that turned into a love match.

THE NEXT THREE months after the wedding, we waited for my Canadian student visa, staying at my uncle's place in New Delhi while I commuted back and forth to the AIIMS for work. Arti was finding out what it was like to be married to a busy doctor. The visa finally arrived, and on March 14, 1975, we took an Air India flight to Ottawa via Rome and Montreal. Because of Indian government regulations, we could only take a minimum of foreign currency. We arrived in Canada with two suitcases and $1,000, courtesy of my father-in-law.

Our plan was to spend only a couple of years here while I upgraded my knowledge and got additional surgical experience. I expected to return to New Delhi to work under Dr. Prakash at the Institute—a considerable risk because he hadn't offered any firm commitment. At the very least, I told myself, we could always go back to Raipur where

I could work with my father as a general surgeon. In the meanwhile, I wanted to make the most of this opportunity.

The landscape couldn't have been more different. I looked out the airport window and saw fresh snow on the ground—not on a distant mountaintop but right there. A beautiful sight to behold. On the other hand, stepping out into the cold with our bags was a complete shock. I shuddered at the frigid blast of air. I was wearing my warmest garb, a nice woollen coat, but Indian woollen coats, I soon realized, have no lining. Welcome to Canada! How on earth would we manage? And how on earth did the people who always lived in this weather manage? I was apprehensive enough about working in a Canadian hospital. Now I had to add this to my worries! We didn't have any money to buy warmer clothes. How long would this weather last? Wasn't spring coming? What would we do?

Then I looked over at Arti. I didn't see any fear or apprehension in her face. Instead, she gazed out a window with a look of intense curiosity. A whole new world for her, something to take in, to learn more about. Not for the first time did I see how right this marriage was and would be. Neither of us ever expected that we would spend the rest of our working lives in Canada, but I had at my side a self-described modern Indian woman, ready to discover—and uncover—something totally different and new.

She turned to me and smiled. Welcome to Canada.

4

A New Beginning

Those first couple of weeks in Ottawa we stayed with Arti's uncle Jack (Jagdish) and Aunt Vini. They had lived in Canada for fifteen years by then. Jack was a scientist at the National Research Council and Vini was an anesthesiologist at a community hospital. How grateful we were for their hospitality and kindness. We stayed in their house while they went away on a previously planned vacation to Florida.

We used public transportation because we had no car or driver's licence between us. More standing out in the cold, waiting for a bus, shivering. The weather was menacing. No wonder her aunt and uncle had gone to Florida.

Soon, though, we moved into a new place where I could walk to work without even going outside. Our new apartment, our very own first rental home, was on the seventh floor of a tall building on Parkdale Avenue near the Ottawa Civic Hospital. Living in a high rise was completely daunting—all those windows and people coming and going by elevator—but the upside was I could get to the hospital by taking the elevator down to the parking garage and then walking through a heated underground tunnel directly to the hospital. My introduction to Canadian ingenuity in dealing with inclement weather.

My salary was $12,000 per year, which seemed like a lot when converted into Indian rupees. But in Canada, it would be just enough for the necessities of life and meager savings for a rainy day—although rain sounded more alluring than the bitter cold. We yearned to talk to our loved ones back in India but even a quick call home, at a dollar a minute, was ruinous.

We made a few short calls, but stuck to written correspondence as much as possible, crowding as much news as we could on the thinnest airmail paper imaginable, writing in very small letters. We waited eagerly for every letter that came from home, while they could not get enough from us. How could we begin to describe where we were and what we were doing? One of the things that continued to startle us was how few people there were, compared to India. Here we were in the capital of Canada and the streets seemed empty by comparison. So much space between the big, wide cars.

We set up house without any household help—another novelty. At least Arti loved exploring this new land. She'd get on the bus and go shopping, even if she bought just a few things. She signed up for a two-year course at an art school, something to do while I was busy at work. Still feeling like a newlywed, I was discovering what an independent-minded, intensely curious woman I had married.

DR. GORDON BEATTIE, chief of general surgery at the Civic Hospital, became my boss and, I hoped, a potential mentor. Tall, well-built, and genial, a true professional, he welcomed me to the division of general surgery. His administrative assistant helped me fill out the reams of paperwork and then introduced me to the staff and showed me around the hospital. The facilities alone had me impressed. Things have changed in India since then, but there was so much here that looked so advanced and up to date—the best in equipment—seemingly taken for granted. I wanted to say, "You have no idea how lucky you are."

My first rotation was two weeks in gastroenterology. Next came cardiac surgery under Dr. Wilbert Keon. How crucial he would become to my training.

In the hospital in Raipur, where I finished my medical school, there was no cardiac surgery. None. At the All India Institute of Medical Sciences in New Delhi, I had a brief rotation in cardiovascular and thoracic surgery. Though the practice of heart surgery intrigued me, a disturbing number of patients undergoing it did not survive. These were mostly adults coping with congenital defects such as a hole in the atrial or ventricular septum, or getting valvular surgery. But even at prestigious AIIMS there was no coronary artery bypass surgery. Not yet. And the head of cardiac surgery there was unspeakably arrogant. We residents were used as second or third assistants in the operating room, to hold retractors and to adjust lights for the surgery. Being yelled at was the price we paid for the opportunity to be in the presence of such supposed royalty.

At the time, rheumatic heart disease was rampant in India and mitral valvular stenosis—a narrowing of the valves—was common. Patients with this condition were operated on without the use of a heart-lung machine, which is meant to take over the jobs of your heart and lungs during surgery, adding oxygen to your blood and pumping the refreshed blood back into your body. Instead, a valve dilator was introduced into the still-beating heart through the left atrium into the mitral valve. The dilator was opened to enlarge the size of the mitral valve and then quickly removed. That was it. Most of these operations were performed by junior staff and senior residents. At least they were nicer to deal with than their superiors. By the end of the rotation, I was delighted when a senior registrar let me do part of the operation. But I also had very little interest in heart surgery. The poor outcomes were too disheartening (excuse the pun).

Dr. Keon, the chief of cardiovascular surgery in the Civic Hospital, was not only superb as a surgeon but also quiet and thoughtful. Quite a contrast to the arrogant doctor I'd had to work under in New Delhi. In India the conventional treatment of coronary artery disease was medical. Cardiologists did not refer patients for any of the surgical approaches at the time—understandable considering the poor results. And as I said, in 1975 in India, there was no coronary artery surgery. Canada was far ahead by comparison. Cardiologists realized the benefit of surgical restoration of blood flow to the heart. Coronary arteries with blockage could be bypassed using a piece of vein removed from the leg. The patient would be on a heart-lung machine and the rates of mortality were low. The results were similarly impressive in the relief of angina.

As a resident rotating through cardiac surgery, I was under the supervision of surgeons and given the duties of looking after patients. The intensive care nurses impressed me with their knowledge and abilities. They were doing tasks that were reserved for junior residents back in India. Seeing how patients were treated with compassion and understanding was a revelation. Such attentiveness and care. I had good basic surgical skills, which served me well in the operating room when called upon to be a second assistant. But this was something new. Hands-on experience in patient management. I soaked it up.

Not surprisingly, the workload was intense. But then, I would not have wanted it any other way. This was what I'd come to Canada for. To learn and grow as much as I could in the few years I'd be here. Poor Arti was discovering what it meant to be married to an absentee husband.

I arrived at the hospital by 6:30 a.m. and left late in the evening. Getting up that early and making my breakfast at a pre-dawn hour was a monumental chore for Arti. Not to mention that cooking—despite her degree in home economics—was a new challenge. Or maybe not exactly "despite" but "because." She'd never been allowed in the kitchen growing up. Nor had I. Earning a college degree was a way to prove that you were meant for other things. I never even washed a dish until we moved to Canada. Surgery wasn't the only hands-on experience I was getting. As Arti would say, she had the recipes for only three dishes: chicken curry, cooked cauliflower, and rice. And that's what she would make.

Breakfast, alas, was the only meal I could be assured of until I came home. Arti could go back to bed after cooking breakfast for me, but I had to go to work. When I got home, I was exhausted. How grateful I was to find a nice hot Indian meal waiting for me, no matter how late. March and April were supposed to be spring months; a glance out the window proved otherwise. The cold stuck around. Fortunately, there was a bus stop right in front of our building. And the buses were heated. What a novelty. Neither of us had ever been on a heated bus. This was a luxury we could afford.

Our weekends were punctuated by a delightful excursion: a bus trip to Sears. There, we immersed ourselves in the lively atmosphere of the department store. And what a culinary treat awaited us at Woolworth's! Indulging in their fish and chips became a welcome respite from cooking for Arti. Meanwhile, as I tended to my hospital duties, Arti's adventurous spirit took her on long bus rides, allowing her to explore the city and satisfy her natural curiosity. It was a simple pleasure, finding joy in discovering a new place.

Fear of failure drove me hard. I was always quick to respond when called by nurses or surgeons. I was continually impressed by the egalitarian attitude in treating patients. There was no pecking order connected to their social status. What mattered was their illness and determining what would be best. I couldn't help but notice how the results of open-heart surgery were very good here; most patients survived. My confidence in the specialty grew.

Despite my fluency in English—all those lessons in school, not to mention my stardom in the elocution contest—there were still occasions when I could not understand local colloquial expressions. I once received a call at 4 a.m., the nurse telling me that a patient had "gone bananas." I asked her to repeat the statement. I then responded, "Well, if she wants one, give it to her!"

With obvious amusement the nurse explained that the patient, who'd had open-heart surgery the day before, was running up and down the corridors like a crazy person. *Going bananas*. Who knew? One more phrase to add to the lexicon.

I was grateful to make long-lasting friends at the hospital, in particular Andrew Pipe who was helpful in sharing the workload and introducing me to the culture of Canada. Andrew was six-foot-five, and we made quite a pair walking up and down the hospital corridors. Mutt and Jeff in white coats. Andrew lent us a transistor radio— remember those?—and Arti and I could switch it on and listen to the world around us, the news, the latest tunes, and an alarm clock that could get me out of bed at an ungodly hour (somehow Arti could go back to sleep after that noise).

Three months in cardiac surgery gave me a good introduction to Canadian medicine. Quite different from the way medicine was practised in India. Like I said, patients came first based on their severity of illness, not on their social standing. And the universal health care system allowed everyone to get good care, regardless of the cost. Universal access to good care—making sure everyone had access to the best—would continue to be a driving factor in my career.

I rotated through general and vascular surgery for three months at a time. I enjoyed the clinical work and got to work more with Dr. Gordon Beattie, the chief of general surgery, who had recruited me for the residency program.

Once, in the outpatient clinic, he asked me to evaluate a patient with enlarged lymph nodes in the neck, something I was quite familiar with from my experience in India. What was my diagnosis, he asked. "Tuberculosis," I said. He seemed genuinely amused and took the occasion to remind me—gently—that tuberculosis was hardly ever seen in Canada. At least not then. He was a good mentor.

The Department of Surgery had an annual resident research day. I was asked to review the charts of patients undergoing parathyroid surgery, and working with a medical student, we presented the work at the research day. We won first prize. Just the sort of news Mother and Father appreciated.

The general surgery rotations were not as labour-intensive as cardiac surgery. I had time to become more familiar with this new country of wide-open spaces and four distinct seasons—spring did finally come with a flush of green and flowers bursting everywhere as well as bright, long summer days. You almost enjoyed it more because you felt you had earned it. Arti and I took the train to Toronto and met some of her relatives there. Weekends were spent with Jack and Vini in Ottawa, getting to know some of their friends.

WHAT BECAME QUICKLY apparent was that we had to get a car, and each of us needed a driver's licence. Driving here was different from

India. First off, you had to drive on the wrong "right" side of the road. Not to mention dealing with snow and the prospect of black ice. Just to make sure she'd do okay, Arti took a driving course with the Canadian Automobile Association. It cost $200 per person: with our limited funds, too expensive for both of us. We bought Jack's 1970 Oldsmobile Cutlass Cruiser for $700. It might have been a bargain, but it sure felt like a bundle.

Once Arti passed the behind-the-wheel test, we were mobile. Now, though, it was my turn. I had driven for years in India and figured I'd be fine on the road in Canada, but then again, I'd heard how difficult the driving test was, especially for foreigners. Most of them failed more than once before passing. A fellow resident at the hospital told me that they were usually easier on doctors. What could I do to prove that I was a doctor? Wear my white coat?

"Carry your voice pager with you," he said. "You're sure to get a call when you're in the middle of the test."

Sure enough, my pager went off while I was driving. "Emergency, Dr. Koshal. Emergency," it shouted.

I recognized my friend's voice immediately and wanted to laugh.

"Are you a doctor?" the examiner asked.

"Yes," I said. My driving test came to an unusually swift conclusion. I passed. I got my licence, just like that. In hindsight, the whole thing was a mistake. I should have taken that driving course. I could have used extra training behind the wheel. Even today I am not as good a driver as Arti is. No false modesty here.

By then we were expecting our first child. We felt settled into a routine of work and home—and not much play for me. That spring of our second year in Canada I was doing my rotation in vascular surgery. In contrast to cardiac surgeons, the vascular surgeons were very slow and methodical. Repair of an aortic aneurysm took six to eight hours. A long day.

On June 11, 1976, I was about to start a long operation with Dr. Neil MacPhail (also known as "MacSnail" for being so slow and meticulous) when Arti paged me. She was having labour pains. I asked her if she could hold off for a while as we had just started surgery. As though Mother Nature would observe this expectant father's command. Clearly, I hadn't spent enough time in obstetrics.

By the time I finished in the operating room, Arti had gotten herself admitted and delivered our first child, Arjun. News that called for more than one long-distance call. Needless to say, both our families were thrilled, as was I. He was the first grandchild in Arti's family, and Arti would be carrying most of the parental load. No Kasturi bai or Sheila bai in Ottawa. Arti would be teaching this child, and all our kids, how to tie their shoelaces almost as soon as they could walk.

Months later, on a weekend, I received a call to inform me that Dr. Beattie had died while playing tennis. I was shocked and devastated. It was a very sad time. I cried at his funeral. Such a loss. He was only fifty-two years old. I had lost my Canadian mentor and worried about my future. What would I be doing now? Returning to India sooner than I thought?

But my future and my career took a curious turn.

DR. KEON, FORMERLY chief of cardiac surgery, took over as chair of the Department of Surgery. When my two years of residency in general surgery were almost up, I'd need to spend another six months in the country to write the Royal College of Physicians and Surgeons exams. I made an appointment with Dr. Keon and asked if I could spend those six months rotating through urology. I was thinking how useful that knowledge would be for me when I went back to India, something I could add to my practice. Dr. Keon had other ideas.

Unbeknownst to me, Dr. Keon had watched me closely during the first three months I was with him. Now he smiled calmly. "I want you to do cardiac surgery," he said. He went on to explain that they were about to start the residency training program for cardiac surgery in Ottawa. He wanted me to be the first resident they took.

I could hardly believe my ears. My initial reaction was to turn him down. The prospect of practising cardiac surgery in India was not alluring, not in the least. What I'd learned already would be good enough. A man of few words, Dr. Keon wasn't going to take no for an answer.

"Young lad," he said, "come back and talk to me in two weeks' time."

Over the next two weeks I talked to a few key people. I soon realized what an amazing offer this was. Evidently, Dr. Keon had been looking for a resident to train for some time. He had a sterling reputation as a mentor, taking good care of his trainees and junior staff. What an honour to be picked. My dilemma was that my parents and colleagues in India, not to mention Arti's family, were expecting me to come back home. Training in cardiac surgery would add to our time in Canada. I hated disappointing my family. And yet, this was an amazing opportunity.

Two weeks later I went back to Dr. Keon's office.

"You will train under me," he said, "and I will train you the way I was trained. After you finish your residency training here, I will send you to Harvard Medical Centre in Boston for a one-year fellowship and then bring you back on staff as a cardiac surgeon. You will be making sixty thousand dollars per year as your initial salary when you become a surgeon."

For a resident who was being paid $20,000 a year and maintaining a family with one son and another on the way, that number—$60,000—was alluring for both Arti and me. But we had to discuss what it entailed. Arti had hoped that now, with my training done, we could relax a little. I warned her that instead, with this stint in cardiac surgery, I would be working harder than ever.

"You need to do this," she said. "It's important for your career."

I looked over at little Arjun and thought, *We need to do this.* It was important for our household and our growing family.

We decided not to tell my parents, at least not for a while. They would be disappointed that we were not returning home. We waited for months, almost a year, before sharing the news. They had mixed emotions, disappointed about our not coming home, but happy that I was advancing my career. My father the surgeon—understandably—took the news better than Mother. Opportunity had knocked.

That meeting with Dr. Keon paved my way for the future in a fashion that I had never imagined. I would have to continue to work as a resident in one of the busiest specialties in medicine as the only resident on that team. The net effect was that I was on call every day, every night, and when I was off, I still came in to work around 6 a.m. and left around maybe nine or ten at night. At times I would be called back in the middle of the night for emergencies in surgery. The prize at the end was that I would be a cardiac surgeon, have an assured income to support my family, and stay in Canada in an elite medical specialty.

There was no written offer or contract. I went with all my trust in Dr. Keon. I sometimes worried about what I would do if, after going through the intensive training, he changed his mind.

There was no turning back. Only looking and moving forward.

5

A Pivotal Decision

Patient rounds at Ottawa Civic Hospital started at 6 a.m. At 7 a.m., the surgeons met in the cardiac surgery intensive care unit for my update on the status of the patients. At the same time, patients scheduled for that day's surgery were wheeled into the operating room. The anesthesiologists would insert the monitoring lines and breathing tube for anesthesia. I would then be called in to start opening the chest.

The attending surgeon, usually Dr. Keon, would come in to place the patient on the heart-lung machine and stop the heart to perform the surgery. The heart would be restarted later using a defibrillator. Once a patient was taken off the heart-lung machine, Dr. Keon would leave, and I would close the chest, stitching up the sternum after it had been opened for surgery. Patients would go into the ICU to recover. I stayed with the patient there until they were stable, checking with the nurses to see if they had any other issues (on alert in case anyone was "going bananas").

Lunch was on the run as I had to be back in the operating room for the next case. Most cases took three to four hours. After the second case, I would go back to the newly admitted patients and write orders, sitting down with a new admission to write a history, do a physical examination, and put down orders for tests and/or medications.

Sometimes there would be a third case or an emergency procedure, which made for a very long day. Exhausting. When I came home, I'd plop myself in front of the TV and turn on Johnny Carson or some episode of *Kojak*, whatever I could find. I didn't really want to watch a show, but I was too tired to talk. Let the TV make noise until I turned to reading a page from the Gita at the end of the day.

I was always on call, but in-house calls—where I was required to be immediately available—were only on alternate days unless there were emergency surgical operations. When on duty, it was hard to sleep because of wake-up calls from the nurses about problems with patients. If I was staying overnight at the hospital, there was a room about the size of a closet where residents could nap. It never lasted long. You'd fall asleep and then hear a nurse's knock at the door. You were lucky to get an hour's sleep. Occasionally we had to take a patient back to the operating room after an earlier surgery for bleeding or other complications.

Every morning the process was repeated. I once had to work on a patient in the operating room for twenty-one hours. It took that long to stabilize the patient. That was the unvarnished truth—the stark reality of the lengths to which one must go to uphold the duty to heal.

On the weekends, after making rounds, I would complete the paperwork for the charts that the surgeons would sign. I took time to read and work on research projects. I couldn't let up. There could be no respite, no easing of the relentless thirst for understanding. The exam that loomed at the culmination of my residency served as a constant spectre, an ever-present reminder of the stakes involved. The mere prospect of failure filled me with profound dread. I had dedicated myself wholeheartedly, and anything short of success would be devastating.

This was one of the toughest times of my life. I thought of it as boot camp—boot camp for the would-be cardiac surgeon. Once, when we were supposed to go to the children's hospital for a case, I went over to Dr. Keon's office and asked his secretary what time we would have to go.

Dr. Keon happened to overhear my question. He barged in and, in no uncertain terms, said, "When you're a cardiac surgeon, you don't care what time it is. You just go." *You just go.* Fateful words.

And go we did.

It wasn't just the lack of sleep that was hard. The challenges extended to the most basic human need: food. Many days I struggled to find an opportunity to eat. You couldn't stop in the middle of surgery for a lunch break and come back later to stitch things up. The cafeteria was only open at midday. If I was lucky, I'd pick up something there for lunch. A slice of pizza was a real luxury. Otherwise, it was whatever I could find in the vending machines—which were not as well stocked in those days as they are today. Cheese and crackers, a bag of chips, some Oreos: the far-from-ideal diet of a cardiac surgeon. The irony was not lost on me, that the very sustenance I consumed amidst the pursuit of healing was far from healthy. Yet, in the whirlwind of my daily routine, the convenience of these options became a necessary compromise. I don't drink coffee. Just tea. I'd make sure I got a cup in the morning and one in the evening. That was it. Occasionally Arti would show up at the hospital with a hot Indian meal for me, which was a particular treat and a source of comfort and support.

I WAS IN the operating room almost every day. This was my life as a resident. I'd come home late, fall into bed, and wake up early the next morning to start it all over again. On the rare occasions when I managed to make it home in time for dinner with the children, Arti would gaze at me with a mix of confusion and concern, questioning what unexpected turn of events had occurred. "Are you okay?" she would inquire, puzzled by my presence during this typically elusive hour.

What kept me going was the promise of a better future for all of us. When I finally became a cardiac surgeon I'd earn a real salary, enough to afford a decent lifestyle in this new country. With this decision to pursue cardiac surgery, it was clear we would not be going back to India. This would be home for our family, the place where our kids would grow up. Yet, the irony was unmistakable. My relentless dedication to my work left little room for the joys of parenthood. The demanding nature of my profession meant that precious moments with our children became rarer. It was a trade-off, a sacrifice required in the relentless pursuit of excellence. And though it weighed on my conscience, I understood it as an inherent consequence of my chosen path, a matter of fact in the pursuit of a brighter future.

Once, when one of our boys was just a school kid, he said to me, as I was darting out, "Daddy, don't go to work." I paused. How would I explain to him that this was what I had to do? This was how we'd pay the bills. "Daddy has to go to work," I said, looking down at the Lego figure he had in his hands. "If I don't, I wouldn't make enough money to buy you toys." He nodded, as if comprehending the trade-offs inherent in our circumstances. Later, he proudly divulged this new-found understanding to his teacher, declaring, "My dad goes to the hospital to make money."

That and to save lives. That would be much harder to explain to a child. How I faced these life-and-death issues every day. It weighed heavily on me. Losing a patient was heartbreaking. We did everything we could, everything that was possible. It was rarer here to lose a patient than it was back in India, which brought a small measure of solace. Still, when I walked through the door at home, I had a hard time focusing on whatever the latest family crisis was, as pressing as it may have been.

Our second son, Anu, was born August 24, 1978, delivered at the Ottawa Civic Hospital. As before, I was unable to leave in the middle of surgery to attend the delivery. Arti arranged a babysitter for Arjun and took a cab to the hospital. Only when we finished up in the operating room was I able to dash over and greet our new-born son. What a joyful sight. His full name, Anurag—he goes by

Anu—means love. I loved my work and I loved my family, and for me the difficult choice was working hard for them when it meant limited time with them.

I remember coming home one night—late as usual—and Arti burst forth with what a hard day she had. She couldn't get one of the boys to eat. Or they hadn't eaten enough. Of course, such a thing could be agonizing, but it posed such a contrast to me having just gone through three gruelling surgeries or spending hours with a patient in the ICU. Arti had to handle so much on her own. I had to remind myself that "not eating enough" was as much of a struggle, and as important in her life, as saving a patient could be in mine.

THE HOURS SPENT within the operating room held a remarkable blend of excitement and rigour. They served as the crucible in which I forged the essential technical skills required for my craft. But a truly exceptional surgeon must possess more than technical prowess alone—they must cultivate the art of clinical judgment. Assisting Dr. Keon gave me the privilege of witnessing a master at work, absorbing his wealth of knowledge and expertise. With each procedure, his calm and composed demeanour remained unwavering, even in the face of the most complex cases. Once his part was complete, when I took charge of closing the chest, his reassuring presence lingered, readily available should the need arise.

At times, I would undertake operations myself, with Dr. Keon assuming the role of my assistant. It was a role reversal for him, accustomed as he was to being the one in charge. Nonetheless, I found solace in the autonomy of working independently, unless confronted with a challenge that I couldn't handle, where his guidance proved indispensable. The countless hours immersed in the operating room were invaluable, surpassing what any textbook could impart. This is where I grasped the true essence of surgical practice, where the art and science converged.

Dr. Keon's success as a surgeon stemmed from his remarkable swiftness and economy of movement. His mastery in minimizing heart stoppage time, also known as ischemic time, was a testament to his skill. With ischemic time typically falling within the range of thirty to thirty-five minutes, he exemplified the principles of a master surgeon: nimble, confident, and precise. The less time the heart was stopped, the better the outcome.

Several years later, a solution called cardioplegia was developed, revolutionizing cardiac surgery. Cardioplegia allowed the heart to be stopped and preserved during the procedure, alleviating the constraints of time and enhancing surgical outcomes. This enabled a broader cohort of surgeons to achieve successful results. Not everyone was a Dr. Keon.

DR. KEON HAD the largest number of patients of all the doctors on staff and dealt with the most complex cases. Some of these took a long time in the operating room. In addition, he carried a large administrative load. He was the director of cardiothoracic surgery, chairman of the Department of Surgery, and the director general of the recently completed Ottawa Heart Institute. A lot of titles meant a lot of responsibility both inside and outside the operating room.

Surgeons are trained by being given graded responsibility in the operating room. First-year residents assist the surgeons. Gradually they are given a non-critical portion of the operation, such as opening the chest, putting the patient on a heart-lung machine, and then, after the major portion of surgery has been done, ensuring control of the bleeding and closing the chest incision. As time goes on, they get to do more and more of the operation. The duration of training varies, as each resident requires a different amount of time to acquire the necessary skills and knowledge to become an independent surgeon. This preparation period allows for a comprehensive and gradual development of expertise, ensuring that each surgeon is fully equipped to handle the complexities of the profession.

Working at the Heart Institute, I was mainly assigned to Dr. Keon but when he wasn't operating, I would assist other surgeons. In a year's span, I took part in over four hundred open-heart operations. Even today I find that number amazing. Here I was, just getting my training, and I was constantly on call, constantly learning. Learning by doing.

As the surgeons became more confident in my abilities and knowledge, they let me do more parts of the operation—under their supervision. At the end of the two-year period, I had garnered extensive experience with some complex cases, such as surgery for an aortic aneurysm or poor ventricular function, or any patient coming in for second- or third-time surgery. Anything that required more than one procedure. More complicated and more time-consuming. I became more and more confident that I would be able to start a clinical practice of my own. Working with different surgeons showed me alternative, interesting approaches to the same procedure, though they mostly followed Dr. Keon's methodology. He set the standard.

I HAD ORIGINALLY come to Canada on a student visa. Now, I would have to leave the country in order to obtain Canadian immigrant status. With a guaranteed job offer from Dr. Keon, I was assured that I'd be able to get a visa back into Canada. Not that I had anything in writing. It was simply what Dr. Keon had promised, and I trusted him. He arranged for me to go to Harvard Medical Centre as a Canadian Heart & Stroke research fellow. I was to work with Dr. Lawrence Cohn, a world-renowned expert in the field of mitral valve repair and replacement surgery, at the Peter Bent Brigham Hospital in Boston— soon to become part of Brigham and Women's Hospital. I'd be mostly focused on medical research, not clinical work.

In July 1979, our little family—Arti, Arjun, Anu, and me—left Ottawa and drove to Boston in our 1970 Oldsmobile Cutlass. It was our first extensive time in the United States. Initially, it didn't look that different from Canada; more buildings, busier streets, huge supermarkets and shopping centres, more people (although nothing like India). The residents were polite enough, maybe a little brusquer than in Canada, but then again, everybody seemed to be in a hurry to get somewhere. I would dress in my usual coat and tie, but these Americans were a lot more casual: blue jeans, sweat-shirts, loafers, parkas.

I was especially concerned about safety in Boston. I'd read alarming news reports about rising crime rates in the States, not to mention the recent riots in South Boston. It all seemed like rampant lawless-ness. I couldn't walk down the street without checking behind me to see if someone was after this short darker-skinned Indian man. Every siren I heard made me fear there'd been some killing—and I was used to hearing sirens around the hospital. We found a nice apart-ment in a good neighbourhood where I could walk to work—alas, not through a heated underground tunnel—and, most importantly, where a security guard sat at the building's entrance. Arti was pleased to discover a nice playground for the kids nearby.

None of this was cheap. The rent was $900 a month in American dollars, and I was making $19,000 a year in Canadian dollars. Not a lot of wiggle room. "At least we won't have to pay Canadian taxes while we're in Boston," I told Arti. But at the end of that calendar year, I checked with the Canadian tax office and was told that, on the contrary, we *would* have to pay taxes.

Financial matters were a huge hurdle for me. In India, when I was growing up, no one ever discussed money. If I needed something, the necessary funds would simply appear. My parents were generous, but they couldn't help us here. As I was trying to figure out what to do—to make pennies fall from heaven—help came in the form of a friend visiting from Ottawa. She happened to work for the Canada Revenue Agency and kindly explained that if I declared my income for when we were in Boston with an accompanying note, we would be fine. She was right. Everything worked out. As always, a good friend paved the way.

Harvard Medical Centre has a well-deserved, long-standing world-wide reputation. I had a year to complete a research project we did in the labs there, testing an alternative to the blood thinners that so many patients had to take. The results, alas, were inconclusive, but then that's what research is for. To learn if something works. It was gratifying to have my paper on the project published in *Circulation*, a prestigious international journal.[4]

With more time on my hands, I went on teaching rounds, even at the Boston Children's Hospital. I met with researchers in cardiac surgery and related subspecialities. What surprised me was the way these top American physicians would address each other and challenge one another, raising their voices to emphasize a point or arguing with their most-esteemed colleagues. I'd never seen that kind of behaviour in the hospitals in Canada, let alone in India. Argumentative, assertive, even combative. One doctor facing another down, waving a finger in the air to make a point. *Why are they being so rude to each other?* I'd wonder. *Somebody's going to get in trouble. Have they no respect?* In time I came to understand that no one took offence. This was normal behaviour, even amongst those at the top of the profession.

The contrasts between Canada and India were evident, but as I ventured into the United States, I realized that it, too, possessed its own unique character distinct from its northern neighbour. Beyond the realm of medical knowledge, I found myself immersed in a cultural education—a valuable complement to my professional growth. For a doctor, effective communication lies at the heart of patient care, and the diverse cultural landscape of North America demanded a keen understanding. Navigating these nuances became an essential part of my journey, enabling me to forge meaningful connections with patients from all walks of life.

Also valuable was having a lot of time to study. There had been precious little opportunity for that in Ottawa since every free moment had been spent in the hospital and the OR. I still had one last exam to pass back in Canada: the Royal College exam in cardiovascular and thoracic surgery. There was so much knowledge I hadn't absorbed or even seen—unlike my Canadian counterparts who'd done much more reading in medical school. I needed to do well on both the written and oral parts of the exam.

I spent countless hours in the Harvard Medical School library, studying intensely, and then flew to Ottawa for the exam. As the time for the exam approached, anxiety took hold. It was an unbearable tension, a cloud of uncertainty that loomed over me. The outcome would remain veiled until a letter arrived in Boston, carrying the verdict of my efforts. "You passed, you passed," I whispered to myself, clinging to a thread of reassurance. There had been no indications to suggest otherwise, yet the weight of the unknown continued to burden my thoughts. In moments of doubt, I drew strength from the teachings I had absorbed from the Gita. It wasn't the end result that held true importance, but rather the act of doing, of pushing forward. I was doing. I would keep doing, regardless of the outcome that awaited me.

During the return flight to Boston, an unexpected announcement jolted me. The pilot's voice crackled over the intercom, signalling a "little problem" that had emerged. Panic gripped me as morbid thoughts of a plane crash and the futility of my relentless study swirled in my mind. The plane, of course, persevered, the issue resolved without us turning back. We touched down safely, my mind a bit more at ease.

A couple of days later, the long-awaited letter arrived, bearing news that cast aside my anxieties. I had passed the exam. It was more a relief than a triumph.

BEFORE RETURNING TO Canada, Arti and I took our two boys and flew to India to see family. "A surgeon," my father had declared. "You will become a surgeon." I had become not only that but a cardiac surgeon. "Why don't you become a brain surgeon or heart surgeon?" Arti had asked when we first met. That had come to pass.

Before we left Boston, we received a crucial letter from Canadian immigration. My papers were ready. All was set. It was a moment of profound relief, a weight lifted from our shoulders. We were on the cusp of becoming landed immigrants in Canada, embarking on a new chapter in our lives within this adopted land. The culmination of years of unwavering dedication and toil was finally yielding its rewards. Everything I had learned and accomplished within the operating room was made possible by the unwavering support and commitment of Arti in our home. Her tireless efforts provided the foundation upon which my own pursuits flourished. The arduous journey we had undertaken was on the verge of reaping its deserved fruits.

Returning to Ottawa held great excitement, especially the prospect of owning our own home with a backyard for the boys to play in—a nostalgic echo of my own childhood. But, of course, with snow for part of the year. And I was now earning $60,000 a year! It might not sound like much now, but in the summer of 1980, that was over three times what we'd been earning. The world was our oyster.

The following year, in anticipation of welcoming a third child into our family, the search for an affordable home began. The prevailing high interest rates and my limited knowledge of the North American housing market left me somewhat uncertain. As always, Arti took charge, diligently conducting the necessary groundwork. My surgical schedule prevented me from actively participating in the house-hunting process. When the opportunity finally arose for me to view a prospective home, I swiftly acquiesced. It felt akin to the acceptance of an arranged marriage, settling for whatever bride my family had chosen. Now, it was a matter of accommodating the desires of this new bride—a quaint house situated in an established neighbourhood on the south side of the city. Three months later, on October 15, 1981, our third son, Amit, was born.

Work continued to be demanding. Except for some weekends, I was mostly an absentee father. I did not know any better. My job was all-consuming. My mentors and teachers had worked tirelessly, and I expected nothing less of myself. The cardiac surgery nurses with whom I spent most of my time treated me with respect and affection. Everyone appreciated my commitment to my patients. I loved what I was doing and thrived on the results of my work.

How else can one go on endlessly, day after day, often without proper meals or sleep?

We rented one house for a year, then we bought a different one, an idyllic, modest home on a quiet tree-lined street. And a mortgage rate of sixteen per cent. *My dad goes to the hospital to make money.* I was afraid I'd have to work forever to pay off that mortgage. But then, at the same time, I took such pride in being able to give my family this perfect place. A cozy bungalow with a large backyard of multicoloured maple, beech, chestnut, and hickory trees that lost all their leaves in the fall and then turned green again in the spring. I was reminded of our yard in India. One year I planted fragrant dahlias beneath the trees, like we had back home. What was I thinking? This was not India. They all died at the first frost. I was better off tending roses like my father did, making sure they were varieties that could survive the brutal winters, or to put it in medical language: choosing ones that had a low morbidity rate.

What took me by surprise was the openness and friendliness of the neighbours, ready to pitch in and help at the least provocation. Like our next-door-neighbour Alex Carman. Almost immediately he perceived how, as a homeowner, I was in over my head. What did I know about yardwork? Back home that was all done by hired help. Not here in Canada. The dads on our block seemed to take pride in their ability to do all those odd jobs around the house, like painting and raking and pounding in nails, not to mention mowing their lawns and shovelling the snow.

The first time it snowed, I tried pushing a shovel around in the mush. Getting nowhere. Alex appeared. "Need a little help with that?" He hardly needed to ask. What did I know about snow? He showed me how to shovel the driveway. Then he picked up a handful of snow, packed it into a ball, and lobbed it over his head. What was that? I was startled. He smiled. My first snowball.

In the warmer weather he helped with the lawnmower, any odd chores I was doing, using a drill for the first time, taking on a bit of carpentry. "Don't I need a circular saw?" I asked. Alex shook his head. Not for what I was trying to do. One gloomy rainy day I figured I'd touch up the paint outside. He rushed over. "No," he exclaimed, "you don't paint in the rain!" Who knew? And the next winter when it snowed, he was the one who helped me push the kids around on a toboggan. Alex will even tell you the story about how he tackled me to the ground when it looked like I would burn my "valuable hands"—his words—trying to use a propane grill.

I was glad to be able to help him when it turned out he needed a repair job on his mitral valve. As a surgeon, it's always difficult to operate on someone you know very well, but in Alex's case—as with others—I thought, *If I don't operate on this friend, I don't want anyone else to.*

Alex had three daughters who could mow and clip or rake in the yard and who ended up being perfect babysitters for our three boys. Arjun was the one who really took to gardening, thrilled to have his first little shovel. What a contrast to my childhood. These boys were growing up Canadian. Being the sole breadwinner with no immediate family close by, I worried about what might happen to them and Arti if anything were to happen to me—not to mention how being a cardiac surgeon offered daily reminders of mortality. I took out life insurance and disability insurance. Arti managed the finances—to my relief—and was careful about our expenses as well as the kids' schooling. She wanted the boys to be active in sports and other extracurricular activities.

We sent them to French immersion schools, good schools with a strong academic record. Living in Canada where fluency in French and English is an asset, the boys would be bilingual—well equipped to thrive in our new country. I had a lot of unilingual French-speaking patients and I often regretted not being able to speak to them in their native language. I'd even made an effort to become fluent by attending some basic French-language courses, but alas, I was so busy I couldn't immerse myself the way our children would. Fortunately, there were plenty of people on staff who could translate for me if necessary. With Ottawa so close to Quebec there had been a push for all of us to be bilingual. I remember sitting in a board meeting when someone made that proposal. Then an influential board member spoke up: "You know, if I need a procedure done, the thing that matters most to me is to be in the hands of the best surgeon around." In the end, everyone else agreed.

Coming back to Ottawa, I had even greater appreciation for how quick and efficient Dr. Keon was with the surgical knife. Those

American surgeons were smart and capable, but much of their time was taken up with giving lectures, travelling, and teaching. By contrast my mentor in Canada was almost always in the operating room, as was I. If you were doing three rigorous surgeries a day, you couldn't help but be efficient, not to mention swift.

In addition to the demands of his surgical practice, Dr. Keon carried a considerable administrative burden that encompassed attending meetings, organizing fundraisers for the Heart Institute, and travelling to conferences. As his trusted associate, I eagerly offered my assistance, immersing myself in the intricacies of his work. Observing and standing by his side proved to be the most invaluable training I could have received.

Years later, when I assumed the role of chief of cardiac surgery in Edmonton, I discovered that the experience and knowledge gained alongside Dr. Keon had prepared me well. I recognized that learning to excel in the operating room was essential, but equally significant was the art of effective administration. Balancing these dual roles was crucial; one could not be pursued at the expense of the other. I embraced the challenge of wearing multiple hats, honing my skills not only as a surgeon but also as an adept administrator. These invaluable lessons equipped me to navigate the complex landscape of my profession, fostering a holistic approach that would prove instrumental in my future endeavours.

6

Boot Camp

W hat follows is an example of what a cardiac surgeon does—a case study, if you will.

Twenty-four-year-old Adam (not his real name) presented to the Ottawa Heart Institute in January 1981 with severe chest discomfort. His blood pressure had fallen, and he was going into shock. With a provisional diagnosis of a ruptured ascending aortic aneurysm, he was rushed into a cardiac operating room.

It was around eight in the evening. I, the youngest (and newly recruited) cardiac surgeon, was called "STAT," which means "Right now, immediately!" Per usual, I happened to be in the building, checking on my patients scheduled for surgery the next morning. I hurried into the operating room just as Adam was being wheeled in.

The place was busy. The anesthesiologist, the perfusionist (responsible for running the heart-lung machine), and the OR nurses had all received the urgent call. Everyone came rushing in at once and quickly changed out of their street clothes and into their green surgical gowns. The patient had a breathing tube and was receiving rapid blood transfusions, procedures that were initiated earlier in the Emergency Room. Efforts at every level to save the young man were in high gear.

Two assistants joined me. We asked the perfusionist to let us know as soon as the heart-lung machine was ready. Time was of the essence. If the aortic rupture was not contained, the patient would die. I opened the sternum while one of the assistants exposed the femoral artery and vein—for access to commence the heart-lung bypass before we opened the pericardium and exposed the aorta and the heart.

When that was done, the patient's blood could be drained through the femoral vein into the heart-lung machine where it would get oxygenated and pumped back through the femoral artery. This was to control blood pressure and oxygenation.

With the patient stabilized, I turned my attention to confirming the diagnosis and repairing the damage. "Has anyone spoken to the family?" I asked.

"He has two older sisters in the waiting room," the nurse coordinator replied, "and they are very worried." Understandably.

"Let them know that we have stabilized him and will keep them informed periodically. He has a major problem with his aorta and the aortic valve is also affected. We will replace the damaged portion of the aorta and replace the valve," I said, just so we'd all be on the same page.

"It will take a few hours and considering how late it is, they might want to go home and rest." I glanced at the clock. "I cannot speak directly to them now but will call them as soon as I am able." I might have been a young cardiac surgeon, but I was already aware of how important it was to reassure any family members. "As you all know, this is a high-risk situation, and we will do our very best. Let them know they can stay in the waiting room as long as they like." No time to pause. "It could be a long night."

With the help of the heart-lung machine, the blood temperature was brought down to 28 degrees Centigrade, or 82.4 degrees Fahrenheit. A clamp was placed on the aorta beyond the aneurysm. The heart was stopped by injecting a solution to protect it. The aneurysm was excised, and the aortic valve was removed. Both of the arteries supplying blood to the heart had to come off the aorta, and they were preserved. An aortic graft and an aortic valve conduit made of animal tissue were used to replace the damaged aorta and aortic valve. The coronary arteries were reattached to the aortic graft. The aortic clamp was removed, and circulation was restored to the heart. The heart started to beat again.

Because of the long time on the heart-lung machine, clotting factors in the blood can get depleted as they go through the machine. In Adam's case there was a significant amount of bleeding. After ensuring that the suture lines were not leaking, it was confirmed that the bleeding was through the graft material used, which was not impervious to blood. This in combination with depletion of clotting factors caused the bleeding. The anesthesiologist ordered clotting factors and the surgeons used local surgical hemostatic agents.

And still the bleeding did not slow down.

By now it was 2 a.m. A message was sent to the family about the status of the patient. Our deep concern was expressed. Despite all our measures, the bleeding continued. A significant amount of the blood was being recovered from the site and pumped back to the patient to maintain hemodynamic stability. Even so, I was worried that the patient might not survive. He went back on the heart-lung machine, we clamped the aorta, and looked inside the graft to double-check that the suture lines were intact. They were. The bleeding was through the semi-porous graft.

Here I was, a fully certified cardiac surgeon doing an operation all on my own, one that called on all my skills, in a situation of dire emergency. After all, the patient was only twenty-four years old. But then, weren't all cardiac surgery situations ones of urgency? Wasn't that what I had already seen?

It was late, but I called Dr. Keon from the operating room (calls in the middle of the night are a hazard of our profession) and explained the situation. He reassured me, letting me know that we'd done—I'd done—all the right things. Still, the bleeding through the graft, which normally stops with these measures, did not abate. More discussion, another late-night call to Dr. Keon. He suggested we rec-lamp the aorta, open the graft, and coat the inside of it with albumin. The danger was that if albumin entered the coronary arteries, the result would be disastrous. This was a last-ditch effort.

We followed his suggestion and carefully avoided albumin going into the coronary arteries and the valve. With the graft successfully closed and the aortic clamp removed, there was a collective sigh of relief as the heart gradually resumed its function. The bleeding subsided over the course of the following hour.

After making sure the bleeding was controlled, we closed the chest. Adam was transferred to the cardiac intensive care unit, and I went out and spoke with the family in the waiting room.

His sisters looked exhausted, fearing the worst. "Everything is okay," I said. I went on to give them a brief overview of the procedure. They were relieved. I warned them that the first forty-eight hours would be crucial, but I was satisfied that we were able to fix the problem.

I went back to see the patient and decided to sleep in the hospital in case of a problem. I desperately needed some rest before operating on my regularly scheduled patient in a few hours. It was 4:30 a.m. I lay down on the sofa in my office and out of sheer exhaustion fell sound asleep. At 6:30 a.m. I woke up and went in to check on Adam. His vital signs were stable but there was still some blood draining through the chest drains. Not surprisingly, his two sisters had not gone home. They were still in the waiting room.

"He's stable now. You can go home and rest. If there is any concern, we will let you know." They were appreciative but did not want to leave the hospital yet.

To be more rested for my upcoming surgeries, I asked the OR to delay my morning case and cancel the afternoon case. I went to the cafeteria and had a much-needed breakfast of eggs and toast with hash browns and a cup of tea. I had not eaten anything since noon the previous day.

The next operation was a straightforward triple coronary bypass that went well. I checked in on all my patients in the hospital, including Adam, and went home.

Arti was concerned about Adam—as she was concerned about all my patients. I told her he was stable. She had made a nice Indian vegetarian meal for dinner. I ate and went to bed. At midnight I got up and called in to check on Adam. He was stable and the bleeding from the drainage chest tubes was slowing down. At last. I went back to sleep.

Adam survived the ordeal and was discharged home after ten days.

IT HAD BEEN fifteen years since I started medical school. All that time of learning, growing, studying, passing exams, and developing my skills had brought me to the next stage in my career. Now at last, I was practising full-time, as a cardiac surgeon in, of all places, Canada. I was a colleague of the very people who had taught me, though they still looked upon me as a junior surgeon. I was young enough, thirty-two years old, and no doubt looked younger. That moustache that had made me look a little more mature to Arti's eyes was still there, in hopes that of commanding respect in my patients' eyes.

I was operating independently, so had to start building up my own referral system. Most patients were referred to Dr. Keon, who would pass a few on to me. Even so, it was not unusual for someone, upon meeting me, to ask if Dr. Keon was going to be in the operating room with me—as though I needed someone else to be in charge. While I continued to help Dr. Keon when he was busy with other issues, when I was operating, neither he or nor anyone else was look-ing over my shoulder. As in the case of Adam, I knew I could always call on Dr. Keon or another surgeon if I needed to: I was on my own but never alone.

Patients came first, and that meant paying attention to whoever came with them, usually loving friends and/or family members, like Adam's sisters, camped out in the waiting room anxiously watching the hours go by.

It was clear to me from the very start how important that was. I'd seen other doctors who left communication with family to other staff members. Not me. I wanted to be sure the patient's loved ones had a chance to meet me, talk to me, ask their questions, get some reassurance and some guidance. You could perform a sur-gery where all went well and then, tragically, the patient died some ten days later. It would be the surgeon who was blamed. Keeping family members fully informed was essential. Even if you had a good meeting with the patient, there can be so much going on in their minds, so many worries and fears, it helps to have family there to talk to. To hear you.

A cardiologist or internist might have a long-standing relationship with a patient, and then a cardiac surgeon comes suddenly into their life, often at a tense, stressful time. All the more reason for the sur-geon to meet with family members and establish a relationship.

My very first cardiac surgical procedure as a consultant, even before Adam, was a patient from the National Defence Medical Centre sent to me by Dr. Fitzgibbon. The operation was a quadruple coronary artery bypass. The operation went well. That night I called in a few times to make sure everything was okay. One of the ICU nurses, realizing how nervous I was, assured me she would call if there was an issue, and I should get some sleep. The patient did well, and this surgeon was very relieved.

I was never without my pager. In this era where everybody has a cellphone in their pocket or purse, it might be hard to imagine the power of the pager, and how essential it was to doctors. About the size of a TV remote control, it went where I went. I'd pat it without even knowing I was doing so, ready to answer anytime day or night. My life in an electrical gadget. Being on call for emergencies—like Adam's—could be especially stressful. The fear of failure was never far off—as always, a motivating force. In time I became more confident and comfortable, but dealing with life-and-death issues is never without apprehension.

And as I said, nor would I want it to be.

Again and again, I'd refer to the Gita, a page or two every night, with passages that remained deeply engrained in my soul. "Work done with anxiety about results is far inferior to work done without such anxiety, in the calm of self-surrender ... They who work selfishly for results are miserable." Such wise words helped me keep a perspective on what I was doing day after day. Cardiac surgery couldn't be more results-oriented, but that is not who I would be in the heat and heart of it. Like everybody else, especially as a newly minted cardiac surgeon, I could be moved by compliments and praise that came my way. But that wasn't who I wanted to be.

Arti helped me here. When I came home and started to go on about the accolades that had come my way, she looked at me very closely and with some disappointment. "Don't come home after a long day and tell me how great you are," she said.

She was so right. It's dangerously easy for a doctor—a heart surgeon especially—to think of yourself as God. You are not. God is God not Dr. Koshal. You are simply doing the best you can and that's good enough. Work is its own reward.

ONE MORNING I was in the outpatient clinic when I got a call from Dr. Keon's office. "Good morning, Dr. Koshal," Susan, his administrative assistant, said. "Dr. Keon is in the operating room and the case will take longer than expected. He is supposed to give a talk at the Rotary Club meeting downtown in an hour and has suggested that you give the talk on his behalf."

"What's he going to talk about?" I asked.

"I'm not exactly sure," Susan said, "but I have a carousel with slides that he was going to use."

I rushed up to the office and picked up the carousel. There must have been over a hundred slides, and I had no idea what was on them. How would I put together a talk and slide show for a Rotary meeting? Another, albeit different, moment of stress.

Susan looked at her watch and said, "Dr. Taylor will be here to pick you up in forty-five minutes." Not much time for prep. "Are you pulling my leg?" I said.

She replied sympathetically, "No."

Dr. Taylor was at the entrance to the Institute, and when he saw me with the slides in hand, there was a clear look of disappointment. He was chief of plastic surgery at the Ottawa Civic Hospital and I knew him well. I explained what had transpired. He explained that the group had been keenly awaiting a presentation by the famous Dr. Keon and the event had been planned for months. I sighed. There was nothing I could do except try my best.

He drove us to the meeting where, brown, scrawny looking, and clutching a slide carousel, I entered a bustling hall filled with Rotarians. I couldn't help but notice the perplexed expressions on their faces. Dr. Taylor took the stage and delivered the news that Dr. Keon could not get out of the operating room and was unable to join. Instead, Dr. Koshal would be presenting. The room seemed to murmur in disappointment.

After lunch and the customary announcements, it was my turn to step up to the podium. Taking in the sea of coats and ties, I couldn't ignore the fact that I stood as the only non-white person in the hall. The first few minutes were crucial—I needed to establish a connection, to bridge the gap and capture their attention. Without planning it, Arvind Koshal, the reputed "best comedian" of his elementary school class, took charge. My inherent sense of humour wasn't about to abandon me in my hour of need.

"Ladies and gentlemen," I said, "I know you were expecting Dr. Keon. Unfortunately, he was unable to leave the operating room. I should inform you that Dr. Keon is my chief, and I am the Indian." There was a short silence, and then laughter and clapping. In that instant, their focus shifted entirely, and I found myself the centre of their undivided attention.

I spoke extempore for forty-five minutes and used only twenty of the slides. My talk focused on the Ottawa Heart Institute and the future of cardiac surgery, things that I cared deeply about, and a topic that I could relate to. No doubt a few of them or friends of theirs had been given a new lease on life thanks to cardiac surgery. A bit of humour from time to time leavened the message. When I finished, I got a big ovation. Dr. Taylor thanked me. He seemed relieved more than anything else.

I wished I could have called my parents then and there. Not for nothing had I learned the art of public speaking back at the Christ Church Boys' High School. Those lessons still came in handy. Knowing how to calmly address an audience, to be confident of your words. This wasn't the "Cataract of Lodore," but a talk at the Rotary Club. Still, "Dashing and flashing and splashing and clashing; / And so never ending, but always descending, / Sounds and motions for ever and ever are blending..."

No prize was awarded but I felt good about how I'd done. Not the results, just the process. Thank you, Reverend Canon J.E. Robinson ... not to mention Robert Southey.

7

Innovations in Cardiac Care

The timing of my arrival at the Ottawa Heart Institute was fortuitous. The practice of cardiac surgery was growing by leaps and bounds. With the introduction of each new procedure and practice, we were able to save more and more lives. That I got to be in on the ground floor, so to speak, was remarkable. When my father dictated, "You will be a surgeon," neither he nor I could have guessed what amazing things I'd be involved with. I'll get to that in a moment. First let me describe some of the other work.

The Ottawa Heart Institute was founded in the mid-1970s, the second in all of Canada (the first was in Montreal, in 1954). One of the biggest advantages of such an institute was that you could have cardiologists and cardiac surgeons working in close quarters. Education, research, and clinical work were brought together all under one roof, enabling greater interaction and cross-fertilization. Ideas could be easily shared, procedures discussed. We could figure out among us the best way to treat a patient. "Patients come first," was not just a feel-good motto. It was how we did things.

In our case, that meant the cardiac catheterization laboratory was across the corridor from the operating rooms. What had to be done in a hurry could be done quickly. A patient could be rushed from one place to the other, if need be. And because we were the Heart Institute, we were empowered to look for new ways to help our cardiac patients.

One of the first things I was asked to do was facilitate a controlled trial in which patients having a heart attack were selected—randomly— to be treated with the conventional medical treatment or to undergo surgery within four hours of the onset of pain. Theoretically, the concept of returning blood flow to a blocked coronary artery in the acute phase of a heart attack made sense, but the logistics of doing so in most hospitals around the world were difficult. But it was something that a dedicated heart institute, like ours, could make happen.

Working with Dr. Don Beanlands, chief of cardiology, and Dr. Keon, a protocol had been established and approved by our Medical Ethics Committee. This meant having surgeons available on most days to operate on short notice and perform an emergency coronary bypass. (Adding to our already heavy workload.) We did it and the results were very encouraging. We presented a summary of our findings at an international cardiology meeting in the United States. The initial evidence suggested that the concept was valid and that immediate restoration of blood flow to the heart was beneficial. The study was published in *Circulation* in 1988.[5]

It was still not feasible to do this in hospitals that were unlike ours until a less invasive way of opening the coronary vessels was made available, such as angioplasty and stenting. Cardiologists could do those in the angiography suite. Indeed, that became the standard of care a few years later. How fortunate we were to be able to explore and instigate the procedure as early as we did.

Starting in 1980, there was a resurgence of interest in cardiac transplantation. With Dr. Keon's encouragement, I attended a congress in the United States to learn more about the challenges of such work. I also dipped deep into the research. The hope was that we could do transplants in Ottawa.

In December 1967, Dr. Christiaan Barnard performed the world's first human heart transplant in Cape Town, South Africa. The procedure was hailed all over the world as a truly amazing feat, which it was. A dying human could now be saved by using a normal beating heart from a recently dead individual. It was a huge, almost unimaginable milestone. Would cardiac surgeons all over the world be able to do the same? Alas, Barnard's patient lived for only a few days and then died from massive acute rejection of the heart. The probability of this occurring to other such patients led to a moratorium on heart transplants.

In subsequent years, continued research and prevention of rejection —or control of rejection—was pursued. What also changed was the definition of death, at least in most of the Western world. Back in Barnard's day, "death" was when the heart stopped beating. But if you were hoping to get a healthy, beating heart for an urgent transplant, that didn't make any sense. "Brain dead," when function in the brain had ceased, became the new criterion for death. By early 1980, there was also strong evidence to show that a combination of the immunosuppressive drug cyclosporine with corticosteroids prevented rejection of transplanted organs, and this led to a resurgence of activity in the heart transplant arena. Of course, the procedure could only be performed as a last resort. With our passion for doing all we could to aid patients, it was only a matter of time before we embarked on a heart transplant. Soon enough in 1984, the time came.

Jean-Guy, forty-three years old, had had two previous heart operations but his heart function had deteriorated, and there was no good surgical or medical option for treatment. His projected life expectancy was about six months. He was placed on the list for transplants. When a suitable donor was identified at the Ottawa General Hospital, the donor was transferred to the Heart Institute.

The surgery itself is not that complicated. With his swift hands and vast experience, Dr. Keon transplanted the donor's heart into Jean-Guy's chest. A first for Ottawa. The media welcomed this groundbreaking procedure. News stories and headlines put us in the limelight. Fortunately, Jean-Guy had an uneventful recovery and left the hospital with a new heart. (He went on to live another twenty-three years—after a second transplant several years later—and became an enthusiastic, regular volunteer at the Institute.)

In those early days of cardiac transplants, there were no established protocols at the Heart Institute. We followed standard criteria that came from the International Society for Heart and

Lung Transplantation to determine who should be a recipient for transplant and how to accept a donor heart. The patient had to be someone with a cardiac problem that couldn't be solved by any of the usual medical or surgical treatments. Most such candidates were not expected to survive six months. We also had to be sure that all their other physical systems were okay: the patient couldn't be suffering from a vast array of other health issues.

As for the donor, they had to be of a similar size as the patient, both in height and weight, and come from a compatible blood group. Once the heart from a donor is taken out, it must be transplanted into the recipient within four hours. This posed a restriction on how far we could travel to obtain such a heart. We had to act fast—but then that was standard operating procedure for our team.

Local donors supplied the hearts for the first few transplants. Still, there were more people needing hearts than were available locally. We needed to expand our reach, seeking out destinations within a two- or three-hour window of flying time. This would give us enough time to remove the heart and transplant it into a recipient within that four-hour limit. The provincial government of Ontario was supportive of the transplant program and with our co-operation they developed the Multiple Organ Retrieval and Exchange Program (MORE). They also provided coordinators for tracking donors and maintaining a list of all possible recipients at different centres.

Our first remote retrieval, in 1984, was to replace the heart in a young eighteen-year-old boy who had had multiple surgeries for congenital heart disease and who was now out of options. He was put on the recipient list. Soon we got a call from MORE that there was a heart available at St. Michael's Hospital in Toronto.

They had done an echocardiogram, reassuring us that the heart was normal. Moreover, the donor's blood group as well as height and weight matched with our recipient. All systems were a go. My friend, the towering—figuratively and literally—Dr. Andrew Pipe, and I were designated to fly to Toronto and retrieve the heart. Because this was a novel situation, the process was filmed for CBC National Television by Terry McKenna. The cameras were on us.

We flew to Toronto on a provincial Learjet, and at St. Michael's Hospital, we removed the heart. From there we were rushed by ambulance to a private hangar, boarding the Learjet with a beer cooler containing a heart wrapped in saline and ice at 4 degrees Centigrade. "I sure hope this works," I said to myself, "because if not, we're going to look like real idiots." Imagine the situation: here we were travelling with a donor heart that had been stopped by us, extracted, and then packed in a polystyrene foam cooler. We expected it to recover and resume function once implanted, but the clock was ticking. Landing in Ottawa, we rushed to the hospital and brought the heart to Dr. Keon, who performed the implant surgery.

There were anxious moments in the operating room. We had to use a defibrillator on the new heart a couple of times before it started to beat. You could feel the tension mounting. The TV cameramen were right outside, ready to broadcast the news. What would we say if things didn't work out? When the heart did restart, we all heaved a huge sigh of relief.

Remote heart retrievals were now added to our arsenal, our bag of techniques, equipment, and medicines. We had to be ready at a moment's notice—beer cooler at hand—when a donor heart became available, flying anywhere in Canada and the United States within that four-hour window of opportunity. And we weren't the only ones. We would find ourselves working side by side with teams from different centres. When a multi-organ donor was available, we would remove the heart, another team would remove the lungs, and another would take the liver. All of this had to be choreographed so that every organ was in good condition, which required enormous co-operation and teamwork. Perhaps that was why a team from Pittsburgh coming to Winnipeg to remove a donor's liver called themselves the Pittsburgh Stealers! But no matter what organ we were taking, we were on the same team.

Our first twenty-five transplants were all successful. Each was extremely labour-intensive, adding to surgeon sleep deprivation. When a donor heart became available, you couldn't just say you'd be there in a couple of days or when more convenient for you. You had to act *now*. No matter how many surgeries you'd done that day.

The outcomes we witnessed were nothing short of invigorating. Suddenly, we found ourselves armed with an additional arsenal of possibilities, offering patients a glimmer of hope and the prospect of a vibrant life that could span many more years—defying the looming spectre of mortality within mere months. Understandably, most transplant recipients were keen to know where the donor heart had come from and whether it was a male or a female organ. Sometimes patients' families wanted to contact the donor family to thank them. However, as noble as these intentions were, a sobering realization dawned upon us: the need for caution in disclosing the donor family's identity without the general agreement of both parties involved. A poignant anecdote springs to mind: a transplant patient, an editor of a newspaper, who took it upon himself to investigate and unearth the identity of his benefactor. Regrettably, he found the wrong person, an example that illustrates the complexities inherent in these delicate matters.

Our initial experience with transplants encouraged us to develop a full-fledged, world- class program. Initially I assisted Dr. Keon in the operating room. Once I was experienced, I performed the procedures on my own, though still under Dr. Keon's name. I was ably assisted by Dr. Roy Masters and Dr. Andrew Pipe.

Dr. Ross Davies became the medical director (cardiac transplantation) and did an outstanding job in identifying suitable recipients and managing them after discharge. Dr. Shiv Jindal who had vast experience in renal transplants, oversaw the anti-rejection regime. We also became part of MORE based in Toronto.

All potential recipients were screened by a team of cardiologists and social workers, and considered at a meeting of the transplant committee, which prioritized them based on the severity of their heart dysfunction and their potential of death. This list was provided to MORE, which had recipients from other Canadian centres and coordinated with United Network for Organ Sharing (UNOS), a parallel program in the United States. International teamwork.

To avoid any conflict of interest, no one involved in the transplant program could be involved in the declaration of brain death of a potential donor. Once brain death was certified, we would be informed, and the team went into action. As usual, the decision as to who received the organ was based on blood group, physical size of the donor, and priority on the recipient waiting list. The transplant cardiologist would be consulted to make the decision. He would also be involved in assessing the quality of the donor heart and recommend tests as required. At the same time, the hospital or unit where the donor was located would maintain bodily functions until the retrieval teams were set to go. It was a matter of life and death, and something that had never been done before. We were all pioneers.

A donor—in the act of dying—can help or even save the lives of many. One donor can potentially donate several organs: a heart, one or both lungs, the liver, one or both kidneys, the corneas, and even bones and skin. However, the orchestration of such a complex process requires the seamless synchronization of specialized teams, each entrusted with the delicate task of procuring their designated organ. In the operating room, the heart received top priority due to the time constraint, followed by the lungs, liver, and, lastly, the kidneys. There could easily be anywhere from two to four different teams, each removing their needed organ. Each team had to be there at the right moment, some coming from other centres in Canada, some from the United States.

The retrieval of a heart from a distant city required meticulous coordination. At the hospital, we ensured that the recipient was anesthetized and ready for the arrival of the donor heart. We used coolers, often purchased from Canadian Tire, to transport the organ. It was crucial to time the procedure precisely, so we refrained from removing the recipient's heart until the donor heart was present and ready for transplantation. Once the donor heart arrived, we initiated the heart-lung machine, removed the patient's failing heart, and carefully implanted the new heart. Time was of the essence as we aimed to complete the entire process, from heart removal to implantation, within the four-hour window.

Within Canada there was an informal understanding that a province would not charge another province for the costs incurred in maintaining a brain-dead donor in the intensive care unit and the use of the hospital operating room facilities. It was not until I received a call from Kentucky, in the US, with an offer of a donor heart that I had any notion of the expense. Per usual, we asked for the necessary tests to assess the function of the heart, which they agreed to.

As I put down the phone, I suddenly wondered, "Will we have to pay for the costs of using their facility?" I called back and they said, yes, we would be billed for everything. The cost would be around US$10,000. I gulped ... and asked for a breakdown of charges. I was told that they divided the costs of maintaining the donor after brain death plus the expense of the operating room among the liver, lungs, and renal teams. And us.

I checked with Dr. Keon, and we agreed that $10,000 was more than we wanted to pay. My next call was to cancel our retrieval. By then, though, they had already done the tests and had organized the retrieval teams for the other organs. I apologized profusely. They agreed to bring the cost down to US$2,000. We went ahead with the transplant.

From then on, Dr. Keon worked with provincial authorities regarding our ability to accept organs from the United States. Thankfully, we received the long-awaited green light, accompanied by the assurance that the associated costs would be covered. It was a pivotal moment that allowed us to transcend borders in our pursuit of life-saving interventions.

This experience, like many others, underscored the stark contrast between medical practices in the two neighbouring countries. In Canada, the notion of crunching budget numbers amidst the throes of a health emergency seemed alien to us. Our focus was firmly rooted in providing the best possible care and saving lives, unencumbered by the financial intricacies that often overshadowed medical decisions elsewhere. The juxtaposition of these divergent approaches was a potent reminder of the profound impact health care systems can have on the delivery of care.

I went on all the initial donor heart retrievals with either Dr. Pipe or Dr. Masters, or sometimes a clinical fellow. Local donors were the easiest to reach due to proximity. For the remote retrievals, MORE would arrange private jets and ambulances for us, anything to minimize the period from stoppage of the donor heart to its implantation. I struggled with airsickness, so my travel preparation included a scopolamine patch on all those flights.

The whole process, starting with the first phone call regarding a potential donor, going to the other hospital, working with various retrieval teams, then removing and bringing the heart back was strenuous. To add to the load, I would assist Dr. Keon and stay until the patient was stable in the post-operative period. Being away from home for long periods of time, not to mention coping with sleep deprivation, was hard. However, seeing a human heart start to beat again in a patient who would otherwise not live much longer—that was unbelievable. You couldn't help being in awe of the results. Even for someone who tried to stay focused on the work not the results, as my Gita reading urged.

The first few transplants generated a lot of excitement in Ottawa. The local press could not contain themselves, and Dr. Keon was widely acclaimed for this accomplishment. In those initial stages, I had the privilege of assisting Dr. Keon during these procedures. Over time, my role evolved, and I assumed the mantle of surgical director for the Heart Transplant Program, ultimately performing the procedures myself.

CONFRONTED WITH THE scarcity of suitable donor organs and the pressing reality of patients in dire need awaiting transplantation, we were compelled to explore alternative avenues. This quest for a lifeline, often referred to as a "bridge to transplantation," aimed to sustain patients' vitality and ensure their survival while awaiting a compatible heart. In pursuit of this goal, Dr. Keon took decisive action and arranged for us to acquire a Jarvik-7, an extraordinary invention hailed as the world's first artificial heart, named in honour of its visionary creator, Robert Jarvik.

The Jarvik-7 consists of two bell-shaped polyurethane pumps that replace the two ventricles, or main pumping chambers, of the human heart. The wide end of each pump is covered with a flexible diaphragm that is blown up with compressed air to expel blood from the chamber and then emptied to draw blood *into* the chamber. The compressed-air power source was a device about the size of a dishwasher that was connected to the Jarvik-7 heart with the machine's ventricles then connected to the patient by tubes. Once it was implanted, it would only keep the patient alive for a few days. As time goes on in these circumstances, the potential for bleeding disorders increases. The procedure could only be a short-term bridge for a patient who was in dire need of a functioning heart and who would not survive otherwise.

Several of us went down to Salt Lake City, Utah, for a three-day training session. We became familiar with how the device worked and shared the information with Dr. Keon on our return to Ottawa. I was asked to develop a consent form and obtain approval for the machine's use in patients from the Ottawa Civic Hospital Ethics Committee. Turning to the consent form used in the first Jarvik-7 implant in the United States, I winnowed down that sixteen-page document to three pages for presentation to the Ethics Committee. After some modifications, it was approved. In the meantime, the cardiac nursing staff, anesthesiologists, cardiac perfusionists, and other ancillary staff underwent in-house training from the manufacturers of the device.

On August 15, 1986, less than a year after the Jarvik-7 had been introduced, forty-one-year-old Noella Leclair was admitted to the Ottawa Heart Institute following a massive heart attack. She had a total blockage of her left main coronary artery, and her left ventricular function was severely compromised, resulting in cardiogenic shock. She was immediately taken to the operating room and placed on the heart-lung machine. I attempted to restore her coronary blood flow by bypassing the blocked vessels with a graft from the saphenous vein in her leg. However, the damage to the heart was severe, and we were unable to wean her off the heart-lung machine. We were informed by MORE that there was no heart donor available.

In the past our patient would have been declared dead. I called Dr. Keon and we felt that her only chance of survival was to use the Jarvik-7 in the hope that we would be able to obtain a suitable donor heart very soon—within the next few days.

We explained the situation to her husband and daughter. We requested their consent to proceed—after all, the Jarvik-7 heart had never been used in Canada before. This was Noella's only chance. A transplant would be sure to give her several more years of life. The family agreed.

Dr. Keon implanted the Jarvik-7. The patient's circulation was restored. With all the material between the artificial heart and the sustaining necessities in her chest, we were unable to close her sternum, but she was alive and connected to this pneumatic compression device by her bedside.

Noella was placed on the most urgent list for donor hearts in Canada as she could only be supported for a few days.

The news of the first total artificial heart implant in Canada at the Ottawa Heart Institute was a big story in the national news. Everyone hoped that a suitable donor would be found soon; someone with a normal heart had to die so that Noella could live.

Noella was kept overnight in the operating room and then transferred, with her chest still open, to the cardiac intensive care unit. It was encouraging to see that she could maintain a reasonable blood pressure on the Jarvik-7. Her kidneys started functioning and her lung function improved on the ventilator. There were issues of bleeding created by the churning of clotting factors with the blood going through the artificial heart. These were corrected. Of course, she required constant minute-by-minute care while we awaited news of a donor heart. Finally, after six anxious days—and sleepless nights— we got the call.

A donor heart was available in London, Ontario. Noella was moved into the operating room in Ottawa, in preparation for the transplant. At the same time, I flew to London accompanied by Drs. Masters and Pipe. The CTV national news team joined us to record the event. Once in London, we removed the donor heart and called Ottawa to give them our estimated time of arrival. We were whisked off by ambulance to a hangar at the London airport where our plane was waiting. We carried the heart with us in a cooler, as we always did. On board the aircraft we were warned that the news had leaked to the press—that we were bringing back the long-anticipated donor heart. Evidently reporters were waiting for us both at the airport and at the entrance to the Heart Institute. With the huge time constraint, we didn't want anything to slow us down. We were focused on getting the heart into the operating room within those four precious hours.

At the Ottawa airport we rushed into a waiting ambulance and managed to avoid the press. But as we reached the entrance to the Heart Institute, we spotted twenty or more reporters milling about. "There's a shortcut we can take," I told my colleagues. We could get to the OR through a side door, well away from the press. We still had the CTV news cameraman and reporter with us, but that was okay. They understood the time crunch.

The ambulance halted at the side door, a mere twenty feet from our destination—the operating room. Yet our progress came to an abrupt halt as a security guard, sternly instructed to prevent unauthorized entry, intercepted us. He demanded to see our photo identification— an expectation we had not prepared for, as we had not anticipated the need to carry our IDs, let alone travel in our surgical scrubs. Standing my ground, despite my diminutive five-foot-five, I explained that we were transporting a heart for a life-saving transplant.

The guard's skepticism was palpable, his retort suggesting he believed our cooler held nothing more than a stash of beer. Realizing that distraction was our only recourse, Andrew Pipe, at his lofty six-foot-five, became the perfect diversion. Engaging the guard in conversation, he skillfully drew his attention, while I seized the opportunity and stealthily slipped past, clutching the precious cargo concealed within the cooler. All the while, the CTV camera dutifully recorded our every move, including this tense encounter.

Successfully delivering the heart to its intended destination, we received a promise from CTV that our confrontation with the guard would not be broadcast on national television. In this high-stakes endeavour, where time and secrecy intertwined, we navigated the labyrinthine landscape of security with a mix of ingenuity, teamwork, and a dash of luck.

Efficient as ever, Dr. Keon removed the Jarvik-7 and transplanted the new heart. We were all overjoyed. The newspapers and TV covered it nationally and the Ottawa media was jubilant.

Noella survived the transplant and lived another twenty years. At almost any other cardiac centre in the world, she would not have survived. At an earlier time, I would have had to walk out of the operating room and convey that sad news to her family. She was fortunate to be in the right place at the right time.

Years later, in 1989, Dr. Keon performed the first neonatal heart transplant in Canada on an eleven-day-old boy, another milestone for the transplant program. The procedure was a success, and the boy, thankfully, lived for many years after.

DURING THE 1970S, the occurrence of death during or after heart surgery was not an unexpected outcome. At that time, we lacked the means to halt the heart for more than a few minutes, perform necessary repairs, and successfully restart it. As a result, the surgeons with the most favourable outcomes were those who could execute procedures swiftly. In each operating room of the Ottawa Heart Institute, a prominent clock resembling a stopwatch adorned the wall, serving as a visual reminder of the fleeting moments. It would be activated when the aorta was clamped, ceasing circulation to the heart, and paused when the clamp was released to restore coronary blood flow. Every minute held profound significance.

Dr. Keon possessed a remarkable efficiency in his movements, completing most surgical procedures within a brief interruption of heart activity. However, if circumstances required more time to complete a repair, restarting the heart became increasingly challenging. Prolonged periods of ischemia caused hearts to become rigid, earning them the evocative label of "stone hearts." Tragically, patients succumbed to this condition.

Researchers at the Heart Institute, as well as other institutions, diligently sought methods to expand the window of time available for successful surgical interventions. It became evident that hypothermia, the deliberate reduction of body temperature, offered some benefits but only to a limited extent. The breakthrough arrived with the introduction of cardioplegia—a technique involving the infusion of a cold solution rich in potassium into the aortic root after clamping. This solution would travel through the coronary circulation, effectively arresting the heart's activity. When combined with localized cooling of the heart and systemic cooling of the patient via the heart-lung machine, it provided a more extended window of time for surgery. Over the ensuing years, the utilization of various additives, including cold blood cardioplegia, facilitated the performance of more complex and lengthy procedures, leading to a considerable reduction in the mortality rate of cardiac surgery.

FOR A SURGEON, losing a patient either in the operating room or shortly thereafter is an indescribable blow. The devastation is profound. After fulfilling the necessary responsibilities such as speaking to family members, completing paperwork, or occasionally contacting the coroner, I would return home. My wife Arti would discern the weight of the situation the moment I stepped through the door. One always questions oneself: could anything have been done differently? Even after more than three decades of performing surgery, the emotional toll of losing a patient remained impossibly heavy. The only solace I could find was in knowing that I had given my utmost effort. Nevertheless, the sense of sadness lingered for days. I had to remind myself that this was an inevitable emotional burden inherent in my line of work. And that's as it should be.

As I told Arti, if I ever *didn't* feel this way after a patient died, I would stop doing surgeries.

8

Go West

When I first met Dr. Keon as a general surgery resident, it took me a while to get used to his manner. I would greet him, with typical Indian politesse, "Good morning, sir!" at the hospital—and hardly get a response. What was I doing wrong? Outside of our intense work relationship in the OR, he barely talked to me for at least two months. Then one morning I was showing him an X-ray and he said, "By the way, you are a very good resident." I was blown away. He cared. He listened. He paid attention. I was doing okay.

At that moment I made a promise to myself that if and when I became a physician with residents working under *me*, I would be sure to be generous with praise where and when it was warranted. It could make such a difference. Despite his commendable qualities, I recognized that Dr. Keon, like many surgeons—including my own father—struggled with moments of arrogance. This trait, albeit not unique to him, occasionally hindered his ability to effectively convey the genuine care and concern he felt for his patients. It served as a reminder of the delicate balance between confidence and humility, and the importance of fostering open and compassionate communication within a sometimes-unforgiving health care system.

Taking note of the valuable lessons we learn is an essential practice. It is through a combination of positive examples and experiences that reveal areas for improvement that we grow and evolve. Dr. Keon, as my mentor, served as a source of both inspiration and opportunities for reflection.

He was a dedicated churchgoer, always attending worship on Sundays, no matter how busy we were. His wife would often bring him around to the hospital afterwards. He'd leave her in the car and launch himself into work. Many times, she could be stuck there for hours, waiting without complaint, as he made rounds. She was a lovely, kind, and, dare I say, incredibly patient woman, the wife of a hard-working surgeon. I was glad when Arti and she became friends. I don't doubt that they commiserated with each other, sharing stories about their absentee husbands.

Working under Dr. Keon, the opportunities for advancement kept coming, with new titles and responsibilities streaming in. I was the first resident trained in cardiac surgery in Ottawa, and then became the program director of cardiovascular and thoracic surgery at the Institute after Dr. Keon. This meant recruiting and training new residents, then participating in post-graduate seminars and supporting research wherever—and when—I could. Once again, I was grateful for that advantage we had in a dedicated heart institute where research, practice, and teaching could all happen under the same roof.

We not only engaged in patient care but also ventured into the realm of research. Through the publication of papers and presentations at national and international forums, we actively spread awareness of our work and its significance. As I advanced in academia, I attained the rank of associate professor, a testament to the collaborative efforts with other researchers, residents, and fellows. Together, we achieved notable milestones. Despite the attention that came my way, I never saw myself as a replacement for Dr. Keon, even if someone had hinted at the unlikely possibility. He was so widely respected and had given me much knowledge and expertise. Only fifteen years my senior, he wasn't a likely candidate for retirement. Not anytime soon.

BY 1991, WE'D been in Ottawa over a dozen years. Our boys were growing and thriving in their schools. We had a house with a backyard. Arti had made good friends. I'd even learned how to shovel snow and mow a lawn—talk about learning new things. Alas, I couldn't really be counted on to know my way from place to place behind the wheel of a car. I'd spent most of my time in Ottawa in one place and one place only: the hospital. If I drove, it was from there to home or from home to there.

I was happy and fulfilled where I was working. Through the different conferences I'd attended I'd come to know other physicians and learned more about what they did—and what they wished they could do. Still, I wasn't looking to move. And I wasn't expecting something else to come along. Certainly not something that might enable me to fulfill my vision for what heart care could become—before I had even fully articulated it.

Then, seemingly all at once, not one but two amazing opportunities knocked at my door. The first came from two cardiac surgeons I was friends with, Dr. Elliot Gelfand and Dr. Dennis Modry, both of whom worked in Edmonton, Alberta. Out of the blue, they issued a formal—and informal—invitation, suggesting that I come and practice there. I wasn't at all sure about the idea. I didn't know much about Edmonton, but in Ottawa, the country's capital and seat of government, distant Alberta had the reputation of being a sort of redneck province. How would a doctor like me—raised in India— fit in? Moreover, how would Arti and the boys fit in? Would we be happy? The whole notion was intimidating. And yet, if I didn't move on somewhere else, I would always be in Dr. Keon's sizable shadow. I needed to think about it. And think about it some more.

After hemming and hawing, I told Dr. Keon about the invitation. He kindly and graciously suggested I should check it out. At the same time, he said he'd like to give me a promotion. When I came back from my visit to Edmonton, he promised he would make me the director of cardiac surgery here in Ottawa. Quite an honour. Clearly, he didn't want me to leave.

I had met Drs. Gelfand and Modry at a conference in Halifax, Nova Scotia, and had enjoyed their company. Gelfand was the clinical head of cardiac surgery and Modry the academic director at the

University of Alberta Hospital in Edmonton. For my visit, they set up an impressive roster of doctors and surgeons from the hospital, as well as the CEO and vice-president of medical affairs. What a daunting lineup.

I flew to Edmonton and the meetings went well, very well. There was a keen desire in the room to have me come and join them. I made it clear—I wasn't just being strategic—that I was happy in Ottawa and would not make a lateral move. It would have to be a promotion. Dr. Garner King, chairman of medicine, took me aside and suggested I put down a wish list of exactly what it would take to make me move to Edmonton.

Back in Ottawa, I sat down with my old friend Andrew Pipe and together we drafted that wish list. It would include: (1) status as full professor and director of cardiac surgery at the University of Alberta, (2) status as clinical head of cardiac surgery at the University of Alberta Hospital, (3) support of the administration in pursuing the building of a heart institute, and (4) development of a ventricular assist program.

The problem was that they would have to give me the positions held by my friends, Drs. Gelfand and Modry, who had invited me to join them in the first place. What would it be like to work in a situation like that? Would they regret even reaching out to me? Maybe the whole thing was preposterous? And yet, I realized I yearned to make the change.

To my delight and surprise, a few weeks later, Arti and I were asked to come back to Edmonton. And then, almost at the same time—like pennies from heaven—I received a call from Winnipeg, from Dr. Blanchard, chairman of surgery, inviting me to come and interview for the position of director and chief of cardiac surgery at the University of Manitoba. Another golden opportunity.

Arti and I visited Winnipeg first and then went on to Edmonton. Both were very persuasive offers. Arti toured Winnipeg while I was being interviewed and liked the city very much. Dr. Blanchard did his best to convince me to come to Winnipeg, but Edmonton still felt like the better offer. The recently built University of Alberta Hospital was a beautiful work environment, full of windows and light. You could come out of the OR and see the sunshine, and the research done within the hospital reflected that same forward-thinking, enlightened approach. Here, they had been pioneers in treating type 1 diabetes with the islet transplant procedure—the Edmonton Protocol—where insulin-producing beta cells, contained in clusters called islets, are isolated from a donor's pancreas, then injected through the skin into the patient's liver. With every conversation I had, I could feel that same interest in expanding all they could do to help treat cardiac patients.

As it turned out, they accepted everything on my wish list.

Back in Ottawa, I worried about sharing the news with Dr. Keon. He didn't hide his displeasure. He even said that he didn't think I would be able to survive—let alone thrive—in a new setting like Edmonton's. I was flummoxed, but I suppose he was accustomed to being in charge: the teacher was not quite willing to give up the student. For whatever reason, not eager to see me leave. He arranged for me to talk to the dean of medicine in Ottawa, who made the formal offer as promised: I would be the director of cardiac surgery if I stayed.

As attractive as that offer was, Arti and I were convinced that it was time to move on. I needed to go it on my own, to spread my wings. And Edmonton, not Winnipeg, would be my new proving ground.

The final meeting with Dr. Keon was excruciating, to say the least. He was unhappy. As though I were rejecting him or was unappreciative of all he had done for me. No words of mine could convince him otherwise. I thanked him again and again for what he had done, giving me this new calling, training me, taking a risk, letting me know I could do what I had never expected to do. He could barely meet my eye. A man of few words at the best of times, he was not going to offer any comfort or reassurance. When I asked him if I'd be able to return to Ottawa if Edmonton didn't work out, he responded briskly, "Once you go there, it's sink or swim." No turning back. As though I shouldn't have even asked. Not long after that meeting, however, his demeanour softened. He and his wife even hosted a wonderful farewell party for me at their home with my parents in attendance.

No doubt about it, leaving Ottawa would be difficult. We had settled in a new country and had developed friends here. This was where I had established myself as a cardiac surgeon. Under Dr. Keon's mentorship, I had the privilege to be part of all the major developments in the field—such as transplantation, artificial assist devices, and surgery in acute myocardial infarction. The fear of failure in a new setting loomed—per usual—but I knew this was an opportunity I couldn't pass up. I turned to my parents, who happened to be visiting at the time. "You need to do this," my father said. They agreed whole-heartedly with me, as painful as it had been to acknowledge how we would not be coming back to India, not to live and work. How our future, and the world of their grandsons, was here in Canada.

First things first, I had to call Dr. Blanchard in Winnipeg, letting him know I had decided to go to Edmonton. What an awkward phone call. I followed that up with a letter, thanking him profusely for his kind hospitality and tempting offer.

All at once the logistics of the move confronted us. We realized that for the boys' schooling we needed to be in Edmonton before the start of the school year. Arti had already looked at some homes in Edmonton—thinking ahead, per usual. She showed me two houses that she liked, and she and I decided on the one we bought and have enjoyed ever since. Decision-making under the gun was not some-thing Arti liked. Neither did I. But there was no other choice. As it turned out, we could move into the house just before the Labour Day weekend. Enough time to get the boys settled before school started and I had to return to work. Because I would be the "boss" at my new job, Arti hoped that my working hours would be more reasonable. What wishful thinking!

All our worldly goods—including our two cars—went into two large moving vans. How startling to see that somehow in the time we'd been here, we'd acquired that much stuff, and couldn't imagine living without it.

The flight from Ottawa to Edmonton was poignant. Saying good-bye to the place that had nurtured us, our first home, the city where Arjun, Anu, and Amit were born. The wonderful people we'd met and the lasting friendships we'd formed. The French immersion schools where the boys had studied and grown, Arti looking after them almost single-handedly allowing me to work long hours—days and nights—in a very demanding specialty.

Despite Dr. Keon's ambivalence about my departure, I would always be grateful for what he'd done for me. Not only passing along the art and craft of cardiac surgery but trusting me enough to represent him at department meetings—giving me the chance to learn whole new skills in management and administration that I would need in this new position. He would candidly discuss administrative issues he was dealing with, giving me an inside look at issues that I would face soon enough. He was good at multi-tasking, helped a bit by the load of work I took on. He'd recently been appointed to the Canadian Senate by the governor general on the advice of Prime Minister Brian Mulroney.

In 1975, we embarked on our Canadian journey, armed with nothing more than a student visa, two suitcases, and a modest sum of one thousand dollars in cash. My initial purpose for coming here was to pursue a residency in general surgery—a path I had envisioned for myself. Little did I know that destiny had something far more remarkable in store. Against all odds, I found myself as the chief of cardiac surgery in a western Canadian city.

A chief, as I liked to joke, not an Indian.

No more looking back. Only moving forward. Elliot Gelfand and Dennis Modry seemed to be okay with me taking over their administrative positions, but I would have to give them confidence that this would be best for all concerned. To alleviate my concerns about Alberta being a "redneck" province, I sought guidance from a trusted friend who hailed from Edmonton. Reassuringly, he dispelled any doubts I had, assuring me that I would not encounter any issues there. In fact, he went so far as to suggest that I might even find a greater sense of comfort and belonging in Alberta compared to Ontario. Soon enough I'd find out.

WE HIT THE ground running. At the top of the Edmonton to-do list: find the right schools for the boys—once again, largely Arti's doing. Arjun was fourteen years old (already!). As in Ottawa, all the boys went to public schools. The Edmonton public school system was and continues to be of high calibre.

We moved into our house shortly after arrival, and Arti and I got settled over the next couple of weeks before I officially started in my new job. As we'd been assured and quickly discovered, the people in Edmonton were warm and welcoming. We were made to feel at home in our new home. I was glad to hear Arti telling her friends back in Ottawa how much she liked Edmonton and how she was well received and embraced. I was intrigued to note how the bilingual culture that had been part of our life back in Ontario didn't seem to exist here. At the hockey games in Ottawa, announcements were made in both French and English; not so here.

I started work in mid-September. The administrative structure in the cardiac surgery department was quite different from what I was used to. There was no single commanding individual, like a Dr. Keon, who could circumvent bureaucracy and make decisions to facilitate care. Cardiac surgery came under the larger Department of Surgery at the hospital, and cardiology under the Department of Medicine. Separate, not joined at the hip—let alone the heart. The academic program of teaching and research came under the chairman of surgery who reported to the dean of medicine, while the clinical program was under the hospital administration. A lot of hoops to jump through.

Again and again, I had to remind myself of the many positives about my new work environment. *You came here for good reason.* The province was flush with money—Alberta is the largest oil and natural gas producer in Canada—and there was the promise of support, from both doctors and administration, to build an excellent heart program. The University of Alberta Hospital building itself was an attractive environment for patients and medical staff alike. The windows and light that so impressed me on my first visit: such a contrast to the tunnel that took me to the hospital in Ottawa. They even had a variety of cafeterias—unlike most hospitals—providing good food for hospital staff and visitors. I would not go hungry, grabbing something to eat in the middle of my crazy schedule.

Looking at a provincial map in relation to our services boggled my mind. The cardiac surgical division served an immense region. The province itself was vast, some 750 miles from north to south and another 400 miles at its widest east-west point. We provided clinical service to Edmonton and nearby areas, such as Red Deer to the south, which was almost a hundred miles away. We also provided services to northern Alberta for adult cardiac surgery, not to mention patients who might come from the neighbouring provinces of Saskatchewan and parts of British Columbia. Open-heart surgery for children was offered for all of Alberta, but there was only one pediatric surgeon on staff. And from everything I saw, the results were not great. So much work to do.

At least they were accustomed to doing heart- and heart-lung transplants at the University Hospital. However, infant transplants were sent to Loma Linda University Children's Health Hospital in California—at a not inconsiderable cost to the province. Only one surgeon did all adult heart and lung transplants. The two adult cardiac surgeons also did some peripheral vascular and lung surgery, but they were transitioning to doing only cardiac surgery. In the meanwhile, a thoracic surgeon had been recruited.

More challenges than I could possibly have imagined. First off, I had to make sure that my two friends, now colleagues, felt comfortable with me taking their leadership positions—something I'd been worried about all along. After all, I was here because of them, and now I feared they would resent inviting me in the first place. I had to be honest with them.

They, in turn, were honest with me.

Apparently, they had been frustrated with the administration as it was. Overworked and under-appreciated, they had all the clinical duties on their plate plus surgeries and emergency calls. Unbeknownst to me, their current appointments were only temporary, unlikely to be maintained for much longer. One of them had even tried to look for another job in the United States, but then realized he was better off in Edmonton. They were grateful not to have to attend countless meetings and deal with the politics to run the division—my new purview. We became good colleagues and would get together with our wives. Good company.

Right off, I established an open-door policy—when I was not in the OR. My colleagues could vent their problems and frustrations with me anytime, and I'm glad they did. We would work together as a team, building excellence and, in due time, a heart institute, God willing.

As in Ottawa, there was a distinguished senior cardiac surgeon on board, Dr. John Callaghan, who had developed the practice of cardiac surgery in Edmonton. A pioneer, he performed the first successful open-heart surgery in Canada in 1956. I was very familiar with his work. During that era, performing successful heart operations posed immense challenges. The heart-lung machine and artificial valves were still in their early stages of development, making each procedure a formidable undertaking. However, the subsequent advancements in technology and a deeper understanding of the heart's response to injury or disease revolutionized the outcomes of cardiac surgery. It was a testament to the progress achieved through improved techniques and increased knowledge. (And this coming from the man who through his dedication to the Gita was determined not to concentrate on results alone!)

Most early heart surgery was done for closure of holes in the septum—at first, atrial septal defect; later, ventricular septal defect and valvular heart disease. Palliative procedures for heart disease were performed without the heart-lung machine for complex congenital heart cases. Surgery for coronary artery disease came in the late 1960s. Dr. Callaghan was also credited as one of the early developers of the cardiac pacemaker—a real game changer.

I was very keen to meet Dr. Callaghan and did so shortly after arrival. Alas, it was a saddening occasion. He was struggling financially and asked me to find some non-surgical work for him so he could make some money. He also wanted me to organize an international meeting to honour him. I suggested a follow-up clinic for patients who had undergone valvular heart surgery; he could use it to collect data for a research project. He agreed to the idea. But goodness, how sad it was to see a man in such distress after years of hard work and innovation. Another note to self: be prepared for retirement. Don't let your ego convince you that just because you are a heart surgeon dealing with life-and-death situations, you can forgo mundane matters like balancing the cheque book and preparing for the future. I vowed that I would never let this happen to us.

The most important issue to address—and change—in Edmonton was the insufferably long wait time patients faced to get heart surgery. Some had waited for over a year and a half. Clearly, an unacceptable state of things. Too many people had developed complications while waiting; some had even died: tragic outcomes that must not be allowed to continue. Some patients were being sent to Calgary or elsewhere to get treated earlier. That couldn't, or shouldn't, have been happening. I would have to find a way to do something.

The obvious solution was to do more surgery—keep things moving apace. Some of it was just a matter of space. The operating rooms, because they were part of the Department of Surgery, were divided between specialties and access was limited. Not only that, but the hospital had a high rate of occupancy with a limited number of beds, especially in intensive care. Almost every patient undergoing open-heart surgery needs an ICU bed. Most can be moved out of intensive care in twenty-four to forty-eight hours, but if there was a lung transplant patient or a complex case with significant post-operative complications, other patients would have reduced access. How would we work around that?

One of the big problems was that the surgeons on staff did only two operations a day. Back in Ottawa, we did two or three. Drawing inspiration from the nimble and deft hands of Dr. Keon, we needed to work swiftly and efficiently. That was also a benefit for the patients. If you moved too slowly, a patient would spend more time on the heart-lung machine. Two hours, as opposed to forty-five minutes, meant longer patient recovery time in ICU.

Within two weeks on the job, I started doing surgery myself. Two or three procedures a day on the days I worked, as I did in Ottawa. The administrative demands of the job would not go away, but I wanted to tackle this problem head-on. Not by telling but by show-ing. I didn't want to be the kind of boss who arrogantly proclaims, "Do it like me." I wanted to offer a model of how things might be speeded up. And anyway, surgeons are a savvy, competitive group. The best of them want to improve. You don't throw down the gauntlet without them picking it up.

The bigger issue turned out to be financial, an administrative snafu. Cardiac surgeons were on a fee-for-service arrangement, and fiercely envied by other doctors for their earning power. Any request for more OR time was seen as a demand for more money, as though the cardiac surgeons were trying to game the system. How could I explain that performing more surgery was essential to reduce the mortality rates and the long wait time? It wasn't about the doctors; it was about the patients. Patients had to come first.

Certainly, I could extend my own hours in the operating room, but I recognized that this alone would not bring about significant change. There were moments when I even considered going to the press, publicizing Edmonton's distressing wait time. There'd be a story to tell. A scandal to make tongues wag. But that short-term thinking would surely backfire on me.

I needed to alert the administration and the powers that be—without any publicity—to get things to change. I talked to the CEO and president, presenting my case, then made a formal presentation to the University of Alberta Hospital board. Tears came to my eyes as I spoke, showing them the dismal statistics.

"There's so much we can do," I said, "to change this." Patients with open-heart surgery didn't need to stay in the hospital for ten days; four or five days would do. What we came up with was an early-discharge program with at-home follow-up by nurses and social workers. "It will help them and help us," I said. We could double the number of surgeries while reducing the need for more beds—a win-win proposition.

To my great relief, the board understood our needs and agreed to our approach. Within months we had significantly reduced the wait time. I came to Edmonton in 1991. It took year after year of focusing on that goal, making progress a little at a time, but in the last few years before I retired in 2013, we got the waiting list down to a week and a half. Only ten days of waiting for elective heart surgery. This was remarkable. We were able to treat more patients faster and more efficiently, saving countless lives.

I didn't have to make some big self-congratulatory speech. The statistics spoke for themselves, and I wanted the world to know. "Look what we've done!" I would say. This time I decided I would go to the press directly to share the good news. What a tremendous difference we were making—it had to be worth publicizing.

The editor I spoke with at the Edmonton paper was cordial, but then she confessed there really was no story. No bold headline to grab readers. Bad news was much easier to sell!

All the more reason to write *this* book.

9

New Challenges

had started as a surgical resident when I first arrived in Canada, and while imperfect, that training was invaluable to me. I wanted to make sure we had a strong residents' training program for cardiac surgery in Edmonton. The residents were not only there to learn—and the surgeons to teach—but also to help us, taking on some of the duties of the surgeons, like checking on patients in the ICU, doing night calls, and sharing the clinical duties. That would free up the surgeons to deal with other issues.

Residents were also key to many of our research projects. You had an idea for a project, and by putting a resident on it, the grunt work was shared. When the results were presented or published in scholarly journals, it was important to ensure that the resident's name was prominently attached to the work. This not only gave them due recognition by adding to their resumé, but also provided them with valuable exposure and publicity. It was a win-win proposition.

That said, to be a resident was a very demanding job. They could be on duty for a twenty-four-hour stretch, like I was. Yes, they were paid, and I promised that when they finished their training—a six-year process—I could guarantee they'd have jobs as cardiac surgeons. Their hard work would not be for naught. We would make sure they had good offers. But a fine residents' program was also a report card for the hospital itself. People noticed. When residents felt they were getting good training and liked the doctors they assisted, they spread the word. More budding surgeons would be keen to apply. The program would rise in esteem within the medical world.

In Ottawa, I'd been all alone, the first and, for a long while, the only resident in cardiac surgery. It was an extraordinary experience, launching me in my career. I received incredible training. I was keen on having something similar for Edmonton, although a little less isolated experience for the resident. I would have been grateful to have a few other residents along for the ride. Cardiac surgery might seem like a place for superstardom, but as I keep insisting, it could never be supremely successful without teamwork. It's what *we*, not I, do. Residents and fellows (doctors training for a subspecialty) were key members of the team.

As I assumed leadership responsibilities, I took the opportunity to assess the state of our residents' program and gain insight into its functioning. To my surprise, I came across an intriguing anomaly. Each year, a celebratory dinner was organized to honour the residents—a tradition observed in many training programs. However, I discovered that a significant number of residents, as they candidly shared with me, chose not to attend these events. It became evident that they felt undervalued and wanted more hands-on surgical experience. And they had concerns about their significance within the program.

This revelation was disconcerting, as it highlighted a gap between the expectations of the residents and the reality of their experiences. It became clear that we needed to address these concerns and bridge this divide. The residents' voices and perspectives were crucial, and it was imperative that they feel valued, supported, and empowered within the program.

To be successful, to put the patients first, Edmonton couldn't be a laggard. We needed a strong program for residents, as well as fellows. We had a couple of good trainees from Canada and others from Puerto Rico, Tunisia, and the United States. It was not uncommon to have residents from across the globe (look at me). But we had to be sure our reputation was such that we would attract the very best.

The upside—and challenge, too—of my open-door policy is that I got to hear both good and bad news. I was gratified that the residents could open up to me, spelling things out face-to face, even as their complaints concerned me. One of the issues involved the physician assistants. The PAs were used to taking over parts of the operations. They felt they deserved priority. But as experienced as they were, if the residents didn't get hands-on experience, they would never develop as surgeons. It was a six-year program for good reason. It took that long—before you added two years for fellowships—to really develop expertise.

That said, some residents could be arrogant. That, too, was unacceptable. Once again, I tried as best I could to offer myself as a model, an example, both as an administrator and as a surgeon on call. During those early days in Edmonton, I was in the OR on an occasion when one of the residents felt the nurse was slow in getting him the instrument he needed. "Same-day service," he snarled. I spoke to him later. "Don't ever address a nurse like that. When you become a cardiac surgeon, you have to set the rules. You can't be rude to the staff. It's unacceptable."

Residents needed to be given priority in the OR. That was the only way they could learn. At the same time, all surgeons were expected to teach. The not-so-hidden agenda of a good residents' program was to replenish the ranks of cardiac surgeons when the older ones were ready to slow down or retire. (This is coming from a cardiac surgeon who made a point of retiring at sixty-five!) We needed new blood and new talent to take up the mantle—or at least put on the surgical gloves and operating gown!

The skills in the operating room are learned through a process of gradual increase in responsibility, step by step. Patient care and well-being should not be compromised. For the first few months, the residents are expected to first- or second-assist a surgeon and are given very little independent operative experience. Over the next months there is a gradual increase in responsibility based on the supervising surgeon's confidence in the resident and their level of expertise. Even after the recommended period of training and obtaining the Royal College certification, most cardiac surgeons need a year or two of Fellowship experience in a subspecialty of their choice, often at another institution. It's a long haul.

In addition to OR experience, residents and fellows needed to develop their clinical judgment, the art and the craft of the practice. It's often more important to know when not to operate than to operate. It's not just a matter of cutting and sewing; a good cardiac surgeon needs to look at the big picture, learning how to make the right diagnosis. No matter how carefully it's done, open-heart surgery is no picnic. It should only be done when necessary. Talking to a patient before surgery, a physician can be tempted to go into a recitation of how successful a cardiac procedure can be, saying something like, "We have a ninety-nine per cent success rate on this" or "We've good experience treating what you're suffering from." All the while, the patient may very well be telling themself, "I'm probably going to be that one per cent failure."

Statistics don't speak to patients. Attentiveness, compassion, and care do, especially at a time of high anxiety. In Ottawa I learned an important lesson, not from Dr. Keon but from a seasoned older gentleman, an experienced plastic surgeon. He gave me a line that I've used again and again with patients. And that I've passed along to our residents and fellows: "The best and easiest thing to tell a patient is, 'Don't worry. We'll fix it. You'll be fine.'" We're there to fix things.

Something else I stressed for the residents and fellows was reading the scholarly medical journals to keep abreast of the most recent developments—there were two or three that were particularly good in our specialty. With the demanding schedule the trainees had, it was easy enough to skip such reading—after all, nobody was going to test them on it. And yet, as a doctor, getting into the regular habit of keeping up with new research is crucial. You discover how the profession is growing. In addition, attending conferences is essential; there were two or three in Canada and the United States that I especially liked. Ideas get shared, new methods trotted out. You also meet fellow cardiac surgeons. How else would I have come to know Dr. Gelfand and Dr. Modry who invited me to come to Edmonton? Learning is something that's ongoing, not just for doctors starting out but for all of us. Establishing that habit right from the start was critical.

The Royal College of Physicians and Surgeons of Canada carries out regular accreditation of the residency programs, a detailed process with external reviewers. Guidelines call for specific objectives in each year of training. At the accreditation review, residents are interviewed and their opinions of their training program carry significant weight—all the more reason to hear out their complaints first within the hospital.

The good news: after our improvements were put into place, making us more attractive to new residents, our program received full approval. In the process we worked hard to ensure that our trainees would pass the Royal College certification exams, both the oral and written parts. How well I remember the stress of those exams when I was a resident in Ottawa. Whatever we could do to make it easier for *our* residents was vital. How gratifying to see us hit a ninety-five per cent success rate.

Those nightly meditations on the Gita helped keep any of this from going to my head. On our flight to Edmonton, Arti had asked me very frankly, "Now that you are going to take on this new job, why don't you become like all the other cardiac surgeons?" I knew exactly what she was saying. Why didn't I make self-congratulation a regular habit? Why didn't I indulge my ego some more? Why didn't I glory in my success? At least it might mean I didn't have to work as hard. I'd be the boss, after all. Who was going to blame me if I didn't answer one of those late-night calls?

I would blame myself.

I'd worked so hard at keeping an open-door policy that it translated to, "Call me whenever you need something, whenever you want to talk." The residents were comfortable sharing with me, at all hours. When they were depressed, anxious, worried, dismayed. They came to know that I wanted them to succeed. Dr. Keon had been a life-changing mentor for me. Now it was my turn. But I would do it differently. With Dr. Keon I'd go for months without getting specific feedback. It was easy enough to interpret his reaction to things as arrogance. Easy enough for any cardiac surgeon to get a little full of themselves. That wasn't who I wanted to be, not as an example and not in leadership.

WITH EDMONTON RISING in the medical world's esteem, I was asked to do a turn as a Royal College examiner myself. It gave me a chance to see how the system worked from the other side. As mentioned earlier, there are two parts to the exam. For the written portion, each

examiner is asked to send a few sample questions—which I did—
and then compose answers for the questions that are accepted, which
would serve as the basis for judging the candidates' responses. Each
essay is scored by two examiners. If there was a significant difference
in the two scores, the chief examiner would review the answer. Naturally, the identity of the candidates is not revealed.

For the oral portion, each candidate is questioned by two examiners—nothing like what my father experienced in England all those
years ago. The examiners must avow that they do not know the
candidate, usually not a problem to accommodate candidates and
examiners from different parts of the country. We all met at the end,
and if any candidate had failed in some way, the examiner responsible had to explain their reasons. The system was fair and unbiased.
No candidate failed without significant discussion and inquiry.

In fact, the one time in my three-year term that a candidate truly
"failed"—to my way of thinking—was when a person had a perfect
score. A little too perfect. The two examiners looking at the written
part of the exam were surprised that the answer was almost identical, word for word, to the model answer. (I've often thought that if
you were going to cheat, wouldn't you try to make your essay at least
slightly different?) That model, like all of them, was written with multiple sources of information and citations, thorough and complete. It
would be unlikely for a single candidate to cover all the bases. There
was a strong suspicion that the system had been breached. The chief
examiner was consulted, and the concern was whether the entire
process had been compromised. Would the examination have to be

repeated for all the candidates? The Royal College was informed, and after deliberation we were asked to continue the exam for all the candidates. The results of one candidate were to be held as "an anomaly in the system." In the end, the candidate was given a passing grade. There was no evidence that unfair means had been used. Just that lingering suspicion.

WHEN WE STARTED training residents, the surgeons were doing everything. We were the cook, the butler, the maid. The surgeon would take care of the patient in the ICU and then return to the OR. No wonder the volume of surgery was so low. It simply wasn't efficient. It was essential to spread the load, and not just by using the residents. To be successful meant more teamwork.

Over time, we were also able to bring in more fellows. Fellowships usually lasted for one year, but then they were renewable. Canadian doctors received priority for residency positions, but fellows could come from around the world. Fellows could be especially useful in the demanding—and time-sensitive—work of retrieving hearts for transplants. We were fortunate in being able to attract and recruit bright, talented, hard-working fellows from across the globe. At one point we had over a dozen trainees from China. Their English generally wasn't strong enough for them to communicate directly with patients, but they were keen to take back to their country what they learned, which included heart transplant procedures.

With all those Chinese doctors who'd worked with us and then returned to China, Arti kept insisting that we should make a trip to see their country and meet up with them. After all, we'd never been there (and Arti, as usual, was keener to travel than I). It took a while, but we finally did go.

What first-class treatment we were given. Those former trainees were kind, courteous, welcoming, great hosts. The only awkward moment came when I asked one of them how their transplant program was going. All at once his English faltered, as though he couldn't remember how to say anything anymore. I didn't know what the problem was because until then, he'd been confident and fluent, showing off the linguistic skills he'd also developed in Canada. Only later did I learn about the controversy—or as some might say, scandal.

Evidently, in China, the enthusiasm for transplants was such that they had taken the step of getting hearts from executed prisoners. Perhaps even hastening the execution of condemned prisoners who happened to be good matches for the patient. At least that was the story that had been circulated.

Arti was appalled, as was I. There was no evidence that any of our trainees had participated in such an unethical practice, and by the time we learned about it—the media catching wind of it and spreading the godawful story (as always, bad news getting the attention)—China had officially banned organ harvesting from condemned prisoners. If it had truly happened with heart transplants, it would certainly not continue. Never again.

IN THIS STORY of medical training and progress, we have good reason to feel heartened and optimistic. Most of the residents and fellows we trained are now successful cardiac surgeons at leading cardiac centres, with some serving as chief of cardiac surgery. Their impact goes beyond our community and helps people in Canada and around the world. They're dedicated to providing excellent patient care, advancing medical knowledge, and mentoring future surgeons. This is not just about leaving a legacy; it's about our shared goal of improving treatment and care for everyone through learning, teaching, and doing.

10

Children's Heart Surgery

Upon my arrival in Edmonton, I was acutely aware of the pressing need to prioritize pediatric cardiac surgery. Saving children's lives: what could be more important?

Back then, in 1991, there were some sixteen heart surgery teaching centres in Canada, and only a handful did pediatric open-heart surgery. Of those, the one in Winnipeg had to be shut down because of a high mortality rate. I was concerned about how Edmonton was doing and what could be improved. More importantly, how the program could make a real difference in Canada. Not just progress, but lasting progress.

I did not have much experience in pediatric surgery, and obviously had much to learn to understand and evaluate the program. As I said, that was something all of us doctors, no matter how experienced, needed to do: learn and grow.

Dr. Keon did the bulk of pediatric surgery in Ottawa, including the first successful infant heart transplant. After I left, they hired a dedicated pediatric cardiac surgeon in Ottawa, but then again there was not a lot of competition in the rest of Canada. For instance, the one pediatric cardiac surgeon in Vancouver only did uncomplicated cases; essentially Montreal and Toronto were the most highly developed to perform complex procedures in children.

Clearly there was a desperate need that Edmonton could fill. We had to up our game.

The program results were a concern. With the small number of cases that came to Edmonton, it had been determined that we couldn't afford two full-time pediatric cardiac surgeons. However, given the rapid development of pediatric cardiac surgery, especially of infants, we needed a recently trained and experienced pediatric surgeon to bring our program up to date. To fill the gap, as a first step I recruited a surgeon to work as both an adult and pediatric surgeon in Edmonton.

With the only pediatric open-heart program in Alberta, patients from as far away as Calgary were referred to us. Still, no infant heart transplants had been done in Edmonton. The Alberta government had arranged that children—often mere infants—requiring this rare procedure could be sent to Loma Linda University Children's Health Hospital in California. This meant moving the family to Loma Linda where the child would have to wait, usually for more than a few days, to undergo surgery. Once a heart donor was identified, the child would be brought in for the transplant. The hospital stay and the post-operative follow-up costs for each procedure averaged over a million dollars. Some local cases were also referred to pediatric centres in Toronto, Montreal, or the Mayo Clinic in Rochester, Minnesota. Quite simply, if we could provide good pediatric surgery, families would not have to take their child out of the province for these procedures, and we would thereby save taxpayer money. This was a win-win proposition.

However, logistics alone weren't our problem. For instance, I learned that one of our sons' classmates, a boy named Ryan, had a complex congenital heart problem. He'd already had surgery once and needed a second procedure. His father was an obstetrician in town and came to my office for advice. He said he would only have the surgery done in Edmonton if I was to do it. I explained that, as a matter of course, I did not perform pediatric surgery. I suggested they try the Mayo Clinic, where Ryan had had a successful operation. The experience shook me: it made me wonder about the lack of confidence in our program.

Then one afternoon the chief of pediatric cardiology in Edmonton walked into my office and closed the door. He was upset about the mortality rate we had in pediatric cardiac surgery. He pointed out that the mortality rate in patients with complex cases, like homograft replacement (using human tissue for an aortic graft), was over fifty per cent. He was deeply concerned, as was I. As he left my office, I assured him that I would investigate the issue. Something had to be done.

When I spoke with the surgeons, they did not feel their results were any worse than those in Toronto or Montreal. They shifted the blame, pointing to inadequate work done by the cardiologists, or the anesthesiologists, not to mention the level of care in the pediatric ICU and on the wards. Only a short while back a similar situation had occurred in Winnipeg's pediatric program. The high mortality rate brought them a lot of newspaper and media coverage. In the end, that program was shut down. That was the last thing I wanted to see happening in Edmonton.

We needed an outside viewpoint. I made a call to the chief of pediatric cardiac surgery at the Hospital for Sick Children in Toronto. I asked if he would come to Edmonton for two weeks, perform surgery while here, and then give me an assessment of what the problem was in our program. He hesitated, saying he was reluctant to do so since he was worried about losing patients in our setting. Clearly, he didn't trust it. Needless to say, I was severely disappointed and worried.

Back in Ottawa, one of our trainees had been Dr. Zohair Al Halees, one of the first residents from Saudi Arabia to work with us. He was now head of a world-renowned congenital heart program at the King Faisal Hospital in Riyadh. Congenital heart disease includes defects that can largely be detected at birth, and his work was a hallmark of pediatric surgery.

I called Zohair and asked if *he* would accept an invitation to come to Edmonton as a visiting professor for two weeks to perform cardiac surgery on children. A man of few words, he readily agreed. He didn't ask for any further details. I was delighted. I thanked him and put the phone down. Then I realized I hadn't said anything about remuneration, nor had he asked.

I called him back and told him that he would be compensated for the surgery he performed, and of course, we'd cover the costs of his travel and stay in Edmonton. Again, the response was, "That's fine."

With the help of our administrative team, we cleared all the red tape for him to work in Edmonton. He came and, over a two-week period, performed sixteen complex pediatric cardiac operations. All the patients survived. And we now had a better idea of where our problems lay. And it wasn't with the cardiologists or the anesthesiologists or the care in the ICU.

Zohair flew back to Saudi Arabia to continue his work. We invited him and a pediatric cardiologist from Los Angeles to perform a detailed review of the pediatric cardiac surgery program and suggest measures to improve. The recommendation was to get a high-calibre pediatric cardiac surgeon. Simple as that.

WHILE THESE EVENTS were taking place, there were changes in the hospital administration with a new CEO and a new vice-president of medical affairs. I was able to convince them of our need for a top-drawer, world-class surgeon. The cost of sending children to other centres was prohibitively expensive. Like that million-dollar price tag to send a child and family to Loma Linda Hospital for a heart transplant. Such a procedure was not only inconvenient for families but also a drain on finances for the entire province. Maintaining a top-notch program here in Edmonton would be a win-win for all.

We were given the go-ahead, and over the next few weeks, I worked with the vice-president of medical affairs to iron out the details. We needed to find the ideal candidate.

Our inquiries and research led us to Dr. Ivan Rebeyka. He had an outstanding reputation for his work at SickKids in Toronto. He was an excellent pediatric cardiac surgeon and, also, had expertise in the Norwood procedure for babies born with hypoplastic left heart syndrome, where their left ventricle and aorta are too small to pump blood to the body. The procedure lets the right ventricle pump blood to the body, a worthwhile alternative to having to do a transplant.

Our pediatric cardiologists thought highly of him and were hoping we could recruit him. He was originally from Saskatchewan and was looking to make an upward move (just the sort of thing I could understand from first-hand experience). We worked on a package that would entice him to come to Edmonton. Ivan was a tough negotiator. In the end, we essentially gave him what he wanted and he accepted the offer.

What a pivotal decision for our pediatric program. Almost immediately there was a big turnaround. We suddenly started getting a surge of complex cases. Very soon a Western Canadian pediatric program was developed and all complex pediatric heart surgery in the west would be done in Edmonton. Some simpler procedures would still be done in Vancouver, but no matter how you looked at it, what we were doing was a huge draw, thanks to Ivan's hard work and talent.

No longer were patients being sent outside of Edmonton for pediatric cardiac surgery. On the contrary, a significant number of referrals were coming *into* Edmonton. Ivan developed an ECMO program for patients to temporarily support the heart and lung function. Much like the heart-lung machine, the technique pumps and oxygenates the patient's blood while the heart recovers. He also used the Berlin Heart, a ventricular assist device for very sick hearts. Edmonton was becoming a centre of training for other programs in North America.

With all the demands on his time and the increased workload, Ivan soon needed another pediatric cardiac surgeon on board, someone who could also instigate an adult congenital heart program, a welcome addition to our surgical division. He suggested Dr. David Ross. David had an excellent reputation as both a surgeon and an individual. He happily accepted our invitation to come to Edmonton and was offered the job.

One little snafu: David also happened to be the only pediatric cardiac surgeon in Halifax. His recruitment triggered a complaint from the premier of Nova Scotia to the prime minister of Canada that Alberta was taking away their sole pediatric surgeon. When the *Globe and Mail* asked me about this, I responded, "Everything is fair in love and hiring." David came of his own accord and felt that this was a good professional move for him. But it was a good reminder how crucial it was to keep training new surgeons to serve *all* of Canada.

Together Ivan and David developed an outstanding program for congenital heart surgery. They handled the most complex cases with excellent survival rates. A tracking system for pediatric cardiac surgery showed that Edmonton now ranked well amongst the best centres in North America. New and better techniques offered hope to many patients considered inoperable in the past. No longer were so many parents facing the tragic circumstance of having to deal with the painful—and premature—loss of a child. Things could be done to help.

That came to include things being done even before a child was born. One of David and Ivan's innovations in Edmonton was developing a successful neonatal heart transplant program. This required a massive team approach with pediatric cardiologists, anesthesiologists, cardiac intensivists, and nurses all working together. Every Tuesday in the newly built auditorium in the Mazankowski Alberta Heart Institute—I'm leaping ahead here—cardiologists from the neighbouring provinces and Calgary would hold a video conference to discuss all of the children's open-heart surgery cases. Decisions would be made regarding treatment. Those patients who required specialized surgery or non-invasive interventions were brought to Edmonton and then transferred back to their respective centres for follow-up care.

There was another helpful and hopeful development. When an adult donor is matched with a recipient, blood group and size matching is usually required. But prominent research pediatric cardiologist Dr. Lori West, who is now at the University of Alberta, demonstrated that infant heart transplants—unlike those for adults—do not require any crossmatching of blood groups because the immune system of infants is still developing. Consequently, when such a patient is diagnosed in utero to have a life-threatening cardiac condition, the baby is placed on the list for access to a donor heart.[6]

At the Heart Institute, when a child with brain death but a normal heart is identified, that donor and the pregnant mother would be brought into two adjacent cardiac operating rooms. The mother would undergo a Caesarean section and in the other room the donor heart would be removed and stored in saline solution at 4 degrees Centigrade. The heart would then be transplanted within a few hours of the birth of the baby with the compromised heart.

As you can imagine, success in cases like this made for interesting reports in national and international newspapers. The loss of one child and the saving of another was poignant for all. And yet many of those parents whose offspring ended up being donors were grateful that the tragic loss they suffered had some benefit—saving a child. I was moved continually by their generosity in agreeing to let their baby offer up a life-saving heart. Since then, more of these cases have been performed. What a welcome turnaround and benefit to the world of congenital heart surgery.

11

Improving Care
in Winnipeg

'd seen how a review by an outsider could greatly benefit a program, spearheading multiple changes and often promoting innovation. Outside experts can draw attention to something that might not be so obvious to (or perhaps be willingly ignored by) others. They can provide the catalyst to make change-for-the-good happen. But it can't simply be a formality. For change to happen, they need to be given authority.

With all medical treatments and services covered by the state, lots can go wrong. Witness that one-and-a-half-year wait time for heart surgery that existed in Edmonton before we made some dramatic changes. That's the sort of critique you often hear levelled at a state-sponsored health care system like the one in Canada. I understand those complaints. But when all patients have access to the same good care, no matter who they are, and all parties work together, medicine is at its best. Without a long wait time for *anyone*.

Let me give you an example of how things went from bad to good in a cardiac program I reviewed. I was grateful to be a part of it.

First, the bad. Fifty-eight-year-old Diane Gorsuch had been on the waiting list for cardiac surgery for over two years in Winnipeg, Manitoba. In the winter of 2003, she died in a shopping mall in Winnipeg while still waiting for surgery. The overall statistics were not good. Between 1999 and February 2003, eleven deaths occurred in patients awaiting heart surgery in Manitoba. Not surprisingly, Diane's death sparked an uproar. The media was all over it. In a country where the government is a key player in medicine, if not the *key* player, there were demands for the immediate resignation of the minister of health, Dave Chomiak, who had been in that position since 1999.

An interesting side note here: when Chomiak was moved from that position to become Manitoba's minister of energy, science and technology in 2004, he had been the longest-serving health minister in Canada up to that time. I think that's a good indication of how stressful a job it could be. A politician in charge of the health and well-being of a province can be held accountable—at least in the press—for all its success and failures. Back then, in 2003, in Manitoba, there was significant room for improvement.

After thirteen days of intense scrutiny, Chomiak publicly announced that I would lead an external review of the program. Another chance to be on the other side of things.

I headed to Manitoba.

Cardiac surgery was being performed in the two main hospitals, the Health Sciences Centre Winnipeg and St. Boniface Hospital.

Within an hour of arriving, it became obvious to me that everyone knew of the problems but were frustrated by the lack of solutions. As I was touring the facilities, I bumped into a senior general surgeon friend. He warned me that there had been previous reviews in Winnipeg; they always seemed to announce a review before an election—at the very least to look good, even if they didn't follow the advice given. I was only too aware of the review of the Winnipeg pediatric heart surgery program done a few years earlier. That review had resulted in the program's closure, leaving behind a trail of uncertainty and apprehension. As I contemplated my role in this new position of reviewer, I couldn't shake off the nagging fear of stumbling into a potential minefield of challenges and consequences.

Almost immediately I told the administrators accompanying me that I would not perform the review until I had a meeting with the minister of health. I wanted to make sure that the political will was in place to implement any recommendations I made. Within half an hour I was in Chomiak's office.

As succinctly as I could, I explained to Chomiak that I was a busy surgeon and would not do this review unless I could be assured that my recommendations would be followed. "This can't just be a political move," I said. "And I'm certainly not doing it for the money." In fact, with all the time I would be expected to spend, it was a money loser. I told him that my team would include heart experts from Alberta and the Ottawa Heart Institute, and we would come up with a clear list of how to improve the Manitoba program. I was confident we could fix the problems with cardiac surgery so that the program would become one of the best in Canada.

Chomiak assured me that he would see that our recommendations were implemented. I made an additional request that I be able to review the program in a year to determine its status. Chomiak readily agreed.

I put together a team with a top administrator from the hospital in Edmonton, a senior cardiac surgeon from Ottawa, our chief of cardiac anesthesiology from Edmonton, and a management consultant to assist in coordinating the review and writing the report.

Over the next few months, we interviewed key players at the two hospitals providing tertiary cardiac care, reviewing the facilities and staff. It was especially disheartening to discover a toxic atmosphere between the anesthesiologists at the two sites. There was also a lack of coordination between staff members, not to mention absence of strong leadership.

Within six months we developed a road map to build a first-class cardiac care program in Manitoba and presented it to Chomiak. He commended us for our work and promised to act immediately on our advice. He had a lot on his plate.

In the report, we came up with forty-two recommendations, including the consolidation of all cardiac surgery at St. Boniface with strong cardiology services maintained at both sites; the immediate recruitment of strong physician leaders for cardiac surgery, cardiology, and cardiac anesthesiology as well as an overall head of a regional cardiac sciences program; and the establishment of a dedicated means of funding to provide long-term sustainable support of the program.

To decrease the unacceptable—and alarming—long wait time, there had to be an immediate increase in the number of cardiac surgeries by at least one hundred cases a year. There would be central management of the waitlist to ensure that all patients were appropriately monitored. And finally, the minister of health—with his own cognition and commitment—would report on the implementation of the recommendations in one year's time. No squirming out of it or postponing it. Chomiak would be held responsible.

Exactly one year later, I went back to Winnipeg and was pleased to learn that they had implemented or were in progress of implementing thirty-nine of the forty-two recommendations. Subsequent reports confirmed the improvement in the outcomes and reduction of waitlists for cardiac surgery with minimal mortality of patients while on the waitlist.

IT GOES WITHOUT saying that looking at cardiac care at another centre—being on the outside looking in—is always instructive. You end up taking in how you're doing at your own home base. For me, it was a chance to confront and inspect my own style of leadership. What was effective, what I needed to do to improve, how would I make the greatest difference?

I'd come to Edmonton with expectations of leadership. I'd seen how Dr. Keon worked and got a feel for what worked for me. I did not want to be a bossy, demanding, full-of-himself administrator and cardiac surgeon. And yet I wanted to make a difference, an impact. I came to see that my own quiet, less self-assertive style had strengths of its own. The more I could give credit to others for what they had done and what they deserved, the more we could do together. And the more effective we'd be.

I thought of how Dr. Keon never went to meetings at the hospital with other surgeons, like the plastic surgeons or general surgeons. It was as though they weren't in the same league. I didn't want to make the same mistake. In Edmonton, cardiac surgery came under the Department of Surgery so I was expected to respond to the chairman of surgery. It was an old system, going back to when there was no such thing as cardiac surgery. We were all in the same boat. If we were going to make any changes and improvements, I had to get to know these doctors. I wanted things to happen in a friendly atmosphere. And so, I went to all the Department of Surgery meetings. I didn't say much of anything—just listened.

I perceived the tensions and jealousies among specialties. People thought that cardiac surgeons wanted to increase their workload just to make more money. I wasn't going to argue directly with that. The one thing I could do was make sure that *I* didn't appear greedy. I made a point of never asking for money for myself. As chief of cardiac surgery, I didn't request a raise. At the University of Alberta, I had the status of full professor with a salary of $9,000 a year; I never asked for more.

In Ottawa, as I've pointed out, I'd seen how effective it could be to have everyone in the same building: cardiologists and cardiac surgeons under the same roof—running into each other in the cafeteria, chatting in the halls; research done at the same place—great minds sharing ideas and approaches. It was creative as well as demanding. In Edmonton, cardiologists came under the Department of Medicine, not with us cardiac surgeons in the Department of Surgery. I'd seen how beneficial it was when the two specialties worked together, but I wouldn't have been successful if I demanded that change immediately. Instead, I also went to the Department of Medicine teaching rounds. Making bonds, building up trust.

We also worked with the city's Royal Alexandra Hospital. I wanted us to be perceived as colleagues, not competitors. At the Royal Alex, they did coronary angiograms; we did open-heart surgery. They proposed to do angioplasty and coronary stents even though there was no cardiac surgery at their facility, which was highly unusual because there was a risk that if the procedure was not successful, the patient could require emergency surgery. In my role as regional director of cardiac sciences in Edmonton, I offered to back them surgically if they had a problem during those procedures as we were only ten minutes away by ambulance. The Royal Alex became one of the first in Canada to perform these procedures without onsite cardiac surgery. We could be most effective delivering cardiac care by sharing the load. Every Friday at 7:30 a.m., we'd go over to the Royal Alex and study the list of surgical referrals. Who needed to be treated first? It was the best way to treat more patients with the shortest wait time. Co-operatively.

Early in my tenure, I had received a call from the Royal Alex about a patient of theirs who'd been waiting two months for surgery. "I'm going to send her to Calgary," the doctor said. I practically screamed, "No, please don't." That would be a terrible blow to us. I circled back to our surgeons and emphasized—once again—how we needed to be ready to pick up their load. Just as they picked up ours. A win-win for both of us.

Some of this is hard to write about because it indeed looks like I'm taking credit for our ultimate success. I'm not. I didn't want people to think of what we were developing as Dr. Koshal's work or Dr. Koshal's vision, the way people would often consider the Heart Institute in Ottawa as Dr. Keon's. It would never come to pass that way. Not here. If anyone else wanted to take credit for our success, that was fine by me. As the Gita, my bedtime reading, says, "You are only entitled to the action, never its fruits." How grateful I was to see those fruits begin to multiply.

12

Ethics in Cardiac Care

The heart is an organ that sustains life, but it also has emotional, symbolic, even romantic and religious implications. The latter influences decisions regarding heart transplants and xenotransplantation (animal-to-human transplants). The ethical implications can be complex.

In my personal sojourn with surgery, there were several ethical issues that posed tough decision-making.

In the summer of 1975, when I was a resident in general surgery in Ottawa. I received a call to see a young patient who was bleeding from his stomach. After review, I ordered a blood transfusion as one of the treatment modalities. The nurse told me that the patient was a Jehovah's Witness and would not accept blood. We were asked to look at other options. I was worried about the patient, but my consultant said we had no choice in this regard even if there was a threat to life.

Later I confirmed that since 1945 the governing body of the Jehovah's Witnesses—the Watchtower Society—banned blood transfusions even in life-threatening situations.[7] If the patient's own blood is pre-deposited (autologous blood), it cannot be used unless it remains in the patient's circulation, such as during open-heart surgery using the heart-lung machine. I also understood that blood products such as red blood cells, white blood cells, platelets, and plasma are forbidden. What is acceptable is the use of fractions of the primary components, such as cryoprecipitate and albumin, if the patient agrees. In those days, open-heart surgery usually required two or more units of blood, hence surgery was not a safe option for Jehovah's Witnessess.

Over the next few years, with improvements in heart-lung bypass machines, there was less destruction of blood cells during surgery, and selected Jehovah's Witness patients were approved and operated upon. In addition to the standard surgical consent, a special form was created indicating that no blood or blood products would be acceptable to the patient.

One unusual referral was a heart transplant for a Jehovah's Witness, something that could only be done without blood transfusion. The patient was discussed at combined medical and surgical transplant rounds and was accepted for surgery. The patient survived the surgery but, unfortunately, died post-operatively.

We learned from the Jehovah's Witness experience: it resulted in not routinely doing transfusions for our other patients, thereby reducing the incidence of any transfusion-related morbidity. Over time, I found that I was the surgeon Jehovah's Witness patients came to. We were both willing to take the life-saving risk. I might not have believed what they believed, but that didn't stop me from wanting to help them. I was flattered that they would put their trust in me.

Another ethical issue came up with the treatment of obese patients. In Canada the official definition of obesity was anyone with a body mass index (BMI) greater than thirty per cent. (Once when I was at a conference and I brought up this figure, a guy from Texas said, "Doctor, that would be most of our patients.") Cardiologists are the ones who recommend a patient for surgery. Initially, they seemed wary about sending over obese patients, but we found we could be just as successful treating them as other patients. Sometimes the length of stay would be longer and recovery more difficult, but they didn't need to be turned away.

Finally, an issue that persists and won't go away with people living longer and thriving and then needing cardiac surgery. That is age. With older patients, how do you determine what they can take? Will they have the strength to undergo surgery and fully recover? Initially, we had rigorous age requirements when it came to transplants. Anybody fifty-five or older was not considered a suitable candidate, and we wouldn't accept a donor heart from anyone over forty-five. But then I remember our chief of cardiology turning fifty and posing the question: why wouldn't he be acceptable for a transplant—if need be? We started looking closer at what made for success in a heart transplant. The issue wasn't necessarily the chronological age of the patient but the *physiological* age. First off, you wanted to make sure the other organs were fine.

Take Ray for an example. Seventy-nine years old, he'd had heart surgery twice already when he came to us, and it was determined what he really needed was a transplant. With hearts in such short supply, how could we possibly put him on our list? But then, at seventy-nine, he was still a healthy, very active man. And yet, it did not seem fair to take a young heart from the donor list and give it to him. But then we asked ourselves—and finally asked him: "What if we found a donor heart that maybe wasn't perfect but could still work for you, would you agree to that?" He did indeed. And such a donor heart came up as an option. My colleague Dennis Modry performed the surgery. The patient was the oldest recipient of a heart transplant. He went on to live another eight years.

I found I had to deal with my own biases when it came to age. A cardiologist called to tell me he was sending me a ninety-year-old woman, a candidate for cardiac surgery. Privately, I had my doubts. But when this vital-looking, very active ninety-year-old walked into my office, I had to change my views. She turned out to be a perfect candidate for surgery. We replaced her aortic valve. A week later she was back on her farm milking cows.

SOME ISSUES HAD to go through the hospital's Ethics Committee. They could be helpful allies for the challenges we faced. In the end, what matters most is to do what's best for the patient.

We had to get their approval before using the Jarvik-7 total artificial heart, a method of keeping a transplant patient alive while awaiting a donor heart. For our presentation to the committee, as mentioned earlier, we came up with our own form after reviewing the sixteen-page consent form that had been used for Barney Clarke, the first recipient of the Jarvik in the United States. We ensured that the next of kin were fully aware of the implications of this technology, which would be the first time it was used in Canada. Our first patient, Noella Leclair, would be essentially dead on the operating table and in most instances would have been declared so. We got the consent from her husband and daughter after explaining to them that this was a bridge to a possible transplant. Noella could be maintained on the Jarvik for no more than seven to ten days. If a donor heart could not be found in that time frame, the treatment would have to be stopped. What difficult decisions for a family to make at a time of considerable distress.

The cost of the Jarvik implantation and the hospital care—at the time—would have been $150,000. If everyone who needed this life-saving device got one, the cost would be equivalent to three Trident submarines, not to mention the budgetary impact it would have on other costly life-saving treatments. There could be no easy answers.

Another time in Edmonton, the hospital Ethics Committee had to consider whether a Down Syndrome patient should receive a heart transplant when there were others without that condition who could benefit from the procedure. Donor hearts were always in short supply. The committee was helpful in exploring the pros and cons of many such situations, but the final decision to go ahead or not would be left to the physicians. Some people thought their emblem should be a hedge not a caduceus—because too often it looked as though they were hedging their bets. But it comes down to choosing the appropriate recipient for a donor heart.

ETHICAL ISSUES ALSO emerged in our research to solve the issue of too few donor hearts. Of course, the best heart to replace someone's failing heart is a human heart, but one possible alternative was to use a heart from a different species, xenotransplants as they're called. When I first came to Edmonton, we explored the idea. A pig heart is almost identical to a human heart. But transplanting cross species without rejection was the challenge.

The good news came when a group from Cambridge, England, developed genetically modified pigs with organs that humans would not reject. Transplanted into humans, it would mean patients would survive. Or so it seemed. I got very excited about the idea. Here was a solution. Whenever we needed a heart, we'd have one. After all, didn't we use bovine and porcine valves for heart surgery? Alas, it was a different thing to use the whole pig heart. You could do the transplant, yes, but it was discovered that pigs have an endogenous virus that is dormant in the host until exposed to human blood. It wasn't going to work. More research had to be done.

Interestingly, I had to give a talk in Saudi Arabia about xenotransplants and what the research had determined to that point. One of our former trainees had invited me to come for a big meeting. Then it occurred to me, how would I talk about pig hearts in front of an audience, especially in a Muslim country? "Just don't use the word 'pig,'" one of my colleagues advised. "Say 'porcine.' And whatever you do, don't show any pictures." I did what he said, but as the research has progressed, especially since my retirement, the issue of using an animal heart in a human is still a problem, and not just in Muslim countries. If the ethical and infection issues could be solved, there is enormous hope of being able to treat hundreds of thousands of patients. As with human transplants, it's not surgery that's a challenge. It's everything around it.

13

Building a
Heart Institute

B y the end of my first decade in Edmonton, the University of
Alberta Hospital and the Stollery Children's Hospital had
become the centre for pediatric heart surgery for all of Alberta,
Saskatchewan, Manitoba, and parts of British Columbia. We were
also the only centre for heart transplants in Alberta, Saskatchewan,
and Manitoba. We remained the only centre for lung transplantation
in Alberta and Saskatchewan. At one time, we performed the largest
number of heart transplants of any hospital in Canada (offering this
to both children and adults).

Our Cardiac Sciences program had established real roots, with
important impact not just in the province but also in the country. I
was especially pleased to be made the regional director. We'd shown
what a difference it made when cardiac surgeons and cardiologists
could work side by side as a team, and our success made a good case
for the value of having cardiac care, research, and education all under

one roof. It was time. We needed the funds and backing to build a separate building, Edmonton's own heart institute.

In 2001, Premier Ralph Klein of Alberta announced government funding of $125 million to build a cardiac centre of excellence in Edmonton. (A similar sum was offered to Calgary to develop a bone and joint institute. However, due to lack of coordination between the orthopedic specialists and the Calgary Regional Health Authority, that money was transferred to building the children's hospital. A reminder to us of how essential it was for everyone to co-operate to get the job done.)

Sheila Weatherill, president and CEO of the Capital Health Authority, the administrative health authority of the Edmonton area, was a strong advocate of the heart institute concept and was instrumental in bringing it to fruition. She put together a great team. An engineering firm and architect were chosen, and the vision of a heart institute in Edmonton was shared. It was finally going to happen.

The excitement and enthusiasm generated in the media was a boon. All the while, we wanted to be sure to do it right, which included learning from others and seeing what would work best. A building was a building, and once it was up and running, it would be ruinously expensive to change our minds. We had to get it right from the start. The architectural firm Kaplan McLaughlin Diaz (KMD) was selected. Their lead architect had designed several heart institutes around the world, and we accompanied him to look at other institutes, to see not only what needed to be done but also, as importantly, what need not be done.

Obviously, one of the places we visited was the Ottawa Heart Institute, all too familiar to me. It had been completed in 1976, with those underground tunnels connecting it to the Civic Hospital. There, the operating rooms were across the corridor from the cardiac catheterization labs, and the cardiac surgical ICU was immediately adjacent to the operating room, allowing a quick transfer of patients between them. A life-saving—not to mention time-saving—convenience. The design itself underscored the co-operative care that we wanted to make happen in Edmonton.

Next, we flew to Ohio to tour the highly esteemed Cleveland Clinic. At the time they were in the process of building a new cardiac facility. Why? Because of the distance that separated the various components of heart care. Back then, some cardiac patients had to use a golf cart from the parking lot to the entrance. I was especially chagrined to note the fast-food chain restaurant serving hamburgers and french fries at the entrance to the hospital. I half-wondered what the—heart healthy?—burgers would say to the banners inside proclaiming that the Cleveland Clinic was the best-rated heart facility in the country.

The Texas Heart Institute in Houston was a brand-new centre. In the foyer was a big statue of Dr. Denton Cooley, a pioneer in cardiac surgery, the person most instrumental in building this facility. Well-deserved status and attention, although it was not something I would ever have wanted. A statue of me? Goodness no! This heart institute was not far from Baylor St. Luke's Hospital, where Dr. Cooley had been trained by Dr. Michael DeBakey before the two had a falling out—an unfortunate parting of the ways of two very talented surgeons. It was an impressive modern facility with ten operating rooms, large intensive care units, and an auditorium with state-of-the-art audiovisual equipment that allowed the staff to communicate with centres around the world. What particularly impressed me were the large glass panels that provided welcome sunlight throughout the building. A feature largely missing in other hospitals, they were a healthy contrast to that fast-food restaurant and a reminder to patients of what they could look forward to after treatment—not to mention the view it offered staff amid stressful work. Our group asked how much this new building had cost. "Ninety million dollars," we were told. US dollars. That intrigued me because I'd been told by our administration that we did not have enough money to build operating rooms in our new building. Well, maybe we did.

On our return to Edmonton, I spoke to a neighbour who was the CEO of one of the largest construction companies in North America, PCL. I wondered out loud: if they had built a facility with ten operating rooms for $90 million in the US, why couldn't we? He thought we should be able to, despite the currency difference and the fact that they did this a few years earlier. I spoke to Sheila, and she agreed. A meeting was arranged with a small group of planners, including Al Olson, an Edmonton-based builder. I made sure some of the naysayers—certain engineers and cost experts—were present, too. Al Olson successfully argued with them. We were told to let the committee know exactly what we needed. In the end, we would have all the operating rooms that were required.

To its initial commitment of $125 million for the heart institute, the Alberta government added a further $23 million to offset an increase in the price of steel. At the same time, a fundraising committee was established under the leadership of Bill Comrie, a leading Edmonton businessman who himself donated $4 million to the cause. The goal was to raise $17 million. Many people donated and actively sought donations—I can't begin to list all their names. I was so grateful to every one of them. JR Shaw of Shaw Cablesystems, took a particular interest and proposed to collect $10 million if the institute were named after Don Mazankowski, a well-known politician from Alberta who at one time was the deputy prime minister under Brian Mulroney's conservative government. JR got the nod from the committee, and I got a remarkable lesson in fundraising.

JR had been based in Edmonton and had built his vast telecommunications empire here, but now lived in Calgary. No matter. His heart—so to speak—was still in Edmonton.

JR showed me how charitable donations can blossom when people have direct interactions with the organization that's soliciting their support. Not to just give someone a brochure or a printout of a well-crafted proposal—but to let them see first-hand what their money would go toward. To that end, JR brought several Calgary businessmen to watch us perform open-heart surgery, to let them see how we were saving lives. After each visit, he asked them to donate to the institute. True to his word, he soon fulfilled his commitment.

That said, there was a problem with the name as he wanted it: Mazankowski Heart Institute. I felt it was important to add "Alberta" to the name because of how the Alberta government had led the way with that initial multi-million-dollar commitment. I brought this up to Sheila and she agreed. But no one wanted to confront the magisterial JR Shaw, especially after all he had done for us. Finally, it was decided that I would go to Calgary with my colleague, pediatric surgeon Ivan Rebeyka, and together we would discuss the issue with JR. We wanted to propose that the centre be called The Mazankowski Alberta Heart Institute.

Ivan and I flew to Calgary for the meeting. We'd had some posters done up showing what the name would look like on the building—very impressive—and showed them to JR. He was polite but went on to say that he should have been told all this before he went out to donors, urging them to give to "The Mazankowski Heart Institute." How would they take this additional change? We understood his quandary. We didn't want him to look bad after all he had done for us. "But if there's no mention of Alberta in the name," I said, "people in the outside world won't know where the institute is located." He pondered this, and then said he would get back to us in a few days. We flew back to Edmonton, our fingers crossed.

A week later, JR conveyed his approval and Alberta was added to the name. JR wanted to make sure that Mazankowski was in big letters and "Alberta Heart Institute" below it in smaller letters. Fine by me, and fine with everybody else.

Mazankowski had retired from politics shortly after I came to Edmonton. Only at this point did I discover how widely respected he was, not just in Alberta but in all parts of the country, even by people from opposing political parties. He and I made some fund-raising trips together to British Columbia and Calgary, and I greatly enjoyed his company. On one occasion, I was present for a cele-bration in honour of Don—affectionately known as "Maz"—on Parliament Hill in Ottawa. Not only were Heart Institute donors and other members of the administration present there but also sev-eral Members of Parliament, all looking to meet him. How unusual to see a retired politician being so honoured by his peers.

Through the fall of 2003, more donations streamed in from across the nation, coast to coast, from Newfoundland to British Columbia. Largely because of Maz.

The intense rivalry between Calgary and Edmonton was a given. Sort of like Houston vs. Dallas in Texas. The Edmonton Oilers vs. the Calgary Flames. Calgary was the business centre, second only to Toronto. Edmonton was sort of the second cousin. It's the capital of the province, but as I've seen, outside of the country, Calgary is much better known and a bigger tourism draw. We had to work hard to defuse any tensions.

Naturally there was significant disappointment in Calgary among people who felt a heart centre should be in their city, but we made our case. Edmonton was already the regional destination for heart and lung transplants and major pediatric heart surgery. Most saw the good sense of building in Edmonton and followed JR's lead: we got some sizable donations from Calgary residents. Mind you, a big dona-tion wouldn't change anyone's place on the waiting list for any sort of treatment. Needs came first. Patients were the focus of all our work and our vision. The enthusiasm for the new centre was contagious—in the best sense of the word. Our target of $17 million was exceeded beyond our wildest dreams. We raised $65 million. The Alberta government (in Canada, health care is administered provincially) also gave significant funds for the construction and future operational costs. We now had over $200 million to make the Mazankowski Alberta Heart Institute a reality. The prospect was thrilling.

THE BUILDING WAS designed as a hospital within the University of Alberta Hospital, connected to the main hospital on most floors to allow for patients and doctors to move from one space to the other seamlessly. One part of the building was structured around the emergency facility, which housed delicate MRI and CT scanners. We had to be especially careful with them during construction, lest they be damaged by any vibrations. The other part was a tower with a massive glass curtain—like the one that so entranced us in Houston. Sunlight was always a healing balm.

There were only eight floors in the building but to connect to the main hospital there was an interstitial space eight feet high between each floor for HVAC and other pipes. The net effect was a sixteen-storey tower.

On the roof of the tower was a helipad to bring in emergency cases. A large elevator—or megavator, as it's called—with enough room to accommodate a patient bed (and respirators, etc., plus staff) could transport a patient from the helipad to the Emergency Room on ground level in twenty-three seconds. Every floor had shelled in space for the future addition of beds or operating rooms. We were looking ahead to potential future needs and wanted to be prepared.

Each patient room would have a view to the outside or to the healing garden inside the building. The healing garden spanned the fourth and fifth floor atrium space and offered a water wall, sculptures, herb garden, and peaceful sitting areas—a welcome and comforting green space any season of the year for patients and staff alike. Documented studies showed how a healing garden like ours could speed the emotional and psychological recovery of patients with an uptick in positive attitudes.

The old intensive care unit, with beds separated by curtains, was replaced so that patients would be in individual rooms. All the gadgetry for intensive care was located in a large room with state-of-the-art monitors and equipment. Each room had a large window to the outside that brightened the rooms with sunlight during the day. This dramatically reduced the "ICU psychosis" described by patients, who lost all concept of time and day or night in dark, artificially lit rooms. The individual rooms also reduced infection rates, preventing cross-infection between patients. Once the patient spaces were looked after, doctors' offices were the last to be completed.

In the basement was ABACUS, a research facility that had dedicated, advanced MRI and other scanners, and echo cardiographic equipment. The immediate proximity of the Institute to the clinical sciences building allowed easy access for research. Above the research facility was the Shaw Auditorium, an interactive one-hundred-seat digital classroom. It was designed to facilitate interaction and collaboration among clinicians and researchers in and beyond the Edmonton area.

Another goal was certification of the Institute as a LEED (Leadership in Energy and Environmental Design) Silver building—not just for our patients but for the larger community. Constructed in 2007, ours was one of the first medical buildings in Canada to qualify for LEED certification, something that is now far more common (and a good thing, too). It had four Eco roofs, with lightweight soil and vegetation on top to aid in heat deflection and storm-water runoff. The three-inch-thick massive glass curtain provided light and insulation reducing heating costs by $1 million a year.

The parking lot for patients was connected by a covered bridge to the Institute. Not far was the LRT (light rail transit) station. Both made it easy for family members to visit.

The Institute was unique in its ability to provide pediatric and adult cardiac care all under one roof. The children's invasive procedures and cardiac surgery would be performed in the new building, with the interconnected floors between it and the Stollery Children's Hospital allowing for a flow of patients back and forth. And eventually, as the need for a dedicated pediatric cardiac intensive care unit arose, there was space for it on the fifth floor of the Institute.

Not only did the Institute provide a nexus for surgery and treatment, but thanks to a donation from Jim Pattison's family, a cardiac wellness and rehabilitation centre was added, along with the funds to operate it. We could help patients get back to their everyday life and selves.

The net result was the largest heart institute in Canada (approximately 600,000 square feet, or larger than ten US football fields), providing both adult and pediatric care under one roof —thanks to the Alberta government and generous donors.

The shovels hit the ground in 2003, and we watched the building take shape with fascination. We planned a gala opening, set the date, but inevitably there were delays and setbacks in construction. No matter. We eventually did have the opening on May 1, 2008. Key government and business leaders were present for the ribbon cutting. Prime Minister Stephen Harper officially opened the Institute.

Our vision was "to provide the best cardiac care, when you need it, and to foster research and education so that heart disease will no longer be the principal cause of death in Canada."

We were fully cognizant that in the pursuit of creating a cutting-edge heart centre, it would be easy to fixate on this edifice that rose from the ground, replete with state-of-the-art technology and architectural marvels. However, it was imperative for us to recognize that the mere construction of a gleaming institute is but the opening act in a far more intricate drama. The true essence of the Heart Institute—the heartbeat, if you will—emanates not from steel and glass, but from the individuals within—those skilled hands that perform surgeries, the inquisitive minds that drive research forward, and the compassionate hearts that care for patients in their most vulnerable moments. Building the Heart Institute was an extraordinary achievement, but it's the dedication, expertise, and unwavering commitment of the people within it that truly breathe life into these structures. We had to ensure that these halls would be perpetually filled with the right people, dedicated not just to the present but also to the future. This is the unwritten prescription for excellence in health care.

A FEW YEARS ago, heart disease dropped to second place—after cancer—as the leading cause of death in Canada. I was so grateful. We were saving lives and it was clearly documented. This milestone was made possible by countless innovations and advanced care across the nation, not to mention lifestyle choices. But the Mazankowski Alberta Heart Institute surely played a role, and I was grateful to be a part of it. Who would have guessed all those years ago, when it was decided that I would be a surgeon when I grew up—and a cardiac surgeon as it turned out, that this was what my life would be? What a gift to me!

14

A Great Honour

I n October 2008, Arti and I were in Goa, India, to attend the wedding of my friend Vijay Gupta's son. In the middle of a formal dinner with a few hundred guests, my mobile phone rang. It was the office of the Governor General of Canada informing me that I had been appointed an Officer of the Order of Canada, one of the highest civilian awards in the country.

I was stunned. I never expected to receive such recognition. The citation read:

> One of our leading cardiac surgeons, Arvind Koshal, has significantly contributed to the advancement of health care in Canada. He has performed innovative techniques that have been adopted across the country and was on the team that conducted the first total heart implant in Canada. He also performed the nation's first implantation of a left ventricular device, a small pump that improves blood flow. As

the chief cardiac surgeon with the Capital Health Authority and the University of Alberta, he has developed its cardiac program into one of the largest in Canada. He has also been instrumental in the creation and development of the Mazankowski Heart Institute, one of the most advanced cardiac care centres in the country.

Two things here: I was not aware that I was the surgeon who had implanted the first left ventricular device (Thoratec) in Canada, not while I was doing it—at Dr. Keon's instruction, per usual. And I was a little amused that they left out "Alberta" in identifying the Mazankowski Alberta Heart Institute. After all my work to make sure the location was in the name!

No matter. I was truly honoured.

The award was invested on April 7, 2010, in Ottawa by Her Excellency the Right Honourable Michaëlle Jean, governor general of Canada. What a proud moment for our family. Everybody was present at the ceremony at Rideau Hall: Arti and our three sons, Arjun, Anu, and Amit.

Dr. Keon, himself a recipient of the same award a few years earlier, called to congratulate me. "Now you don't have to prove yourself anymore," he said. How well he knew me. That inner drive was always there, fuelled by a fear of failure and tempered by my nightly Gita practice reminding me that it wasn't the results that mattered. The action was what counted, not the fruits of my labour. Didn't that prove true again and again? The work itself was so rewarding.

I was sixty-two years old and felt I should start planning for retirement. The thought gave me chills and a strange feeling ... of relief maybe. I knew plenty of doctors who had no desire to ever give up. They'd die with their boots on, or at least their surgical gloves on. That wasn't me. But for decades now my professional life had overtaken all other priorities. If or when I had any free time—a rarity—I spent it with Arti and the boys. Even then, I could be called away on some emergency.

The boys had done well in their studies——at college, university, professional schools, graduate schools—and in their careers. Those pursuits had taken them far afield, from Edmonton to Kingston, Toronto, Montreal, the United States, and the United Kingdom. They seemed to have the same drive that I had even as their mother, who largely raised them, helped guide and encourage them along the way. They had made visits with us back to India, but they were Canadian to the core. We loved seeing them, but it was hard to get the whole family together in one place. It took something like that awards ceremony.

Amit, our youngest son, has a PhD in finance from MIT, and he assured me that we would be fine financially if I wanted to retire early. But I wasn't quite ready. I needed time for the transition and to confirm my comfort level. Not to mention preparing my colleagues for my absence (I liked to think they would miss me). I would leave at age sixty-five. The message from friends who had retired was to be sure that I had other things to do. Arti had long been accustomed to my absence during the day and often at night, so I didn't want to be a burden to her. Like that old line, "For richer, for poorer but not for lunch!" Sometimes not for dinner either.

My slew of responsibilities at work included being the clinical director of the Regional Cardiac Sciences program as well as the senior medical director and public face of the Heart Institute. After four terms as director of cardiac surgery at the University of Alberta, I was unlikely to continue in that position. At the University of Alberta Hospital, I was the site chief of cardiac surgery. All the while, I maintained an active clinical practice, including night calls, which were onerous. Instead of dumping those on my fellow colleagues, I arranged to have a senior fellow, Dr. Nitin Ghorpade, a fully trained cardiac surgeon, help with my clinical work. What a welcome addition. He did an excellent job.

Looking back to when I had moved to Edmonton, it was so rewarding to see how far we had come. The appalling over-a-year wait time for elective open-heart surgery had shrunk to two weeks, and by the time I left, it was just a week and a half. There was a healthy decline in morbidity and mortality. We had developed a world-class pediatric cardiac program and performed the largest number of heart transplants of any centre in the country. And as I've said, we had built the largest heart institute in Canada with both adult and pediatric cardiac surgery under one roof. As a nexus of research and education—not just clinical care—we attracted doctors from all over the world for advanced training.

Our success far exceeded my wildest dreams. I had short-term targets of one or two years, but the years all bunched together. How had the time gone so fast? Even after all these years, the possibility of failure was still my biggest motivator, making me work hard and push myself—anything to preserve my reputation (whether or not it might have ever suffered). I wanted my family to be proud of me and to follow the same principles. Indeed, my sons did and continue to do so.

Serving with different mentors in India and Canada, I strived to learn from not just their strengths but also their weaknesses. Dr. Keon worked harder than anyone I had ever met. The ability to multi-task and handle each area in an efficient manner was a characteristic that I watched carefully. He was a busy cardiac surgeon, chief of cardiac surgery, founder and director general of the Ottawa Heart Institute, chairman of the Department of Surgery, and a senator. He could do all this because he performed cardiac surgery expeditiously and had good assistance in the hospital to take care of his patients in and out of the operating room, something I took note of.

Dr. Keon trusted me in the day-to-day work, but also involved me with important events, such as the heart transplant program and the artificial heart implantation. In the operating room, once the patient was stable, he would leave me on my own to finish the procedure, but would be there within minutes if I ran into trouble—something I made sure to do with my trainees.

The most important skill in cardiac surgery is to make appropriate judgment calls at all stages of patient care. I spent long hours in the operating room and the ICU, hardly seeing the light of day (in winter especially, that was quite a change from India). The operating rooms and the intensive care unit were in the basement in Ottawa; access to food was minimal and nil after hours. Which we kept in mind when planning the new building in Edmonton. I had to constantly remind myself that there was light at the end of the tunnel. In more ways than one.

ARTI THOUGHT SHE would see more of me after I completed my training at Harvard and returned to Ottawa, but fresh responsibilities made that impossible. New titles were further added—surgical director of the heart transplant program and director of the residency training program—which gave me local and national recognition. When invited to other centres, out of loyalty to Dr. Keon and the comfortable cocoon of living in Ottawa, I turned down all the offers. Until I finally succumbed to the invitation from Edmonton.

As I've said, Arti has always been tremendously supportive of my work, carrying the bulk of the family load. Anything I could do to help her I was only too glad to do. In Edmonton, she was part of a women's group of medical wives. They were getting together at our house one day to hear a talk about the artist Frida Kahlo. Arti wanted me to get a movie about Kahlo, which I did and then loaded into our video player the night before, trying to make things as easy as possible. All she had to do was press a button.

The next morning, I was in the OR in the middle of an operation. We'd just stopped the patient's heart and the clock was ticking … when I got a message: "Your wife is on the phone. She needs to talk to you right away." I feared the worst. Some accident with the kids or whatever. Ever the efficient multi-tasking cardiac surgeon, I said: "Put her through." There must have been five or six people in the room: the perfusionist, anesthesiologist, two nurses in scrubs—one to bring me the instruments I needed—and at least one orderly. Everybody could hear as Arti said in frustration, "I can't get this darn thing to work!" I knew immediately what she was talking about. "Just point the remote at the DVD," I said, "and click it." At once there was clapping in the background. The video worked. And my colleagues did their best not to tease me about it forever afterward!

Arti was always afraid of the sight of blood and, understandably, had no compulsion to watch an operation. But a couple of years before I retired, she decided—at a friend's urging—that she wanted to see me in action. Usually, we didn't allow anyone else in the OR but this was a special case. After checking that the rest of the team—the anesthesiologist, the perfusionist, and the others—didn't mind, I made it possible. That day I was doing a coronary bypass surgery and replacing an aortic valve. Arti stood at the back where I tried to ensure she could see everything. All of a sudden I heard her ask, "Aren't you going to test that valve before you put it in?" Of course, I couldn't answer. Not then. *Explain later*, I thought. Then as we were sewing up the aorta, clearly thinking she saw spaces between the sutures: "You can see the gaps in there," she said. "Isn't that going to bleed?" I shook my head. No gaps. Everything normal. *Talk later*, I thought.

The rest of the team was blessedly silent. Arti now had a better idea of what my days were like—and in a way, I gained a better understanding of her. That innate curiosity that enabled her to leave our native country and establish a new, richly satisfying life where we were, extended even to confronting her own fears—her squeamishness about blood—and asking questions in the middle of an open-heart surgery. That's my wife: inquisitive, intrepid, unflappable. Qualities I admired, as a spouse and a surgeon turned administrator.

THE VISION OF a heart institute like the one in Ottawa was the driving force in my approach to my work. My surgical colleagues were supportive. I had an open-door policy and assured them of fair treatment. There was a need to work together co-operatively and collaboratively. Any internal issues between them would stay within and be handled within the division. I was fortunate to achieve their trust and support. They understood that everyone would benefit from success. The administration was convinced of our intent to provide the best of cardiac care.

A critical development was the establishment of the Regional Cardiac Sciences program and my selection as director. Not even the premier of the province would deliver the heart institute without wide support at all levels—of the hospital administration and the four other hospitals in the province. A buy-in from everyone was essential. We gave permission to the Royal Alexandra Hospital to perform angioplasty without in-house cardiac surgery, offering backup surgical support at the University Hospital if needed. That went both ways, with coronary care units at all hospitals. I was grateful for the support they gave.

If you don't care who gets the credit, the project will be success-ful. It was we, not me. We needed approval from the Capital Health Authority and Sheila Weatherill, who was convinced of the benefit of a heart institute. The premier would make the ultimate decision, but communication would first have to go through the deputy min-ister of health. I had a good discussion with Shelley Ewart-Johnson. She showed a keen interest in the concept. Unbeknownst to me, she was on a long flight with Premier Klein soon after our discussion and made a strong case to him.

Good things happen that you have no way of controlling or plan-ning—and you might not even learn of them until long after the fact.

I knew I had to make our case to the minister of health, Gary Mar, but wasn't sure how best to reach him. I mentioned this to a politically well-connected friend, wondering if he could arrange a meeting. An hour later I got a call from the minister's office inviting me to breakfast the next day. It turned out to be just the two of us in his office, a one-on-one meeting. I laid out the plan for the heart institute and assured him that, if approved, it could be part of his legacy. "I would love to be part of such a project," he replied.

A few weeks later I was at a function where I got an opportunity to see Premier Klein face to face. In a few short, well-practiced sen-tences I made my pitch, outlining the benefits a heart institute would have for Alberta and how we would make him proud of champi-oning this venture. In 2001, ten years after I came to Edmonton, Premier Klein announced $125 million for a cardiac centre of excel-lence in Edmonton. Victory.

But it wasn't just mine to claim. The support of my colleagues was crucial, particularly Dr. Dennis Modry, who had a close relationship with the premier. Sheila Weatherill was a steadfast believer and used her superior administrative skills to take the project to its completion despite challenges. The support of the University Hospital Foundation and the business leaders across the country was invaluable. Interestingly, some who were initially opposed to the project came around. A few of them even took credit for it.

It is extremely important to have good secretarial and administrative support. In Ottawa, Evelyn Fry was of great assistance, loyal and efficient. When I moved to Edmonton, Edith Hutcheson took over that role. As my administrative responsibilities grew, she single-handedly managed my clinical practice, billings, and all the work organizing meetings, dealing with patients and surgeons, and more. She had a calm demeanour and tended to all these issues while I was busy. I never heard a complaint about her; quite the contrary, everyone who dealt with Edith was pleased and satisfied. She was totally dependable. It made my work so much easier. I was grateful for her dedication and support.

AT AGE SIXTY-FIVE, I decided to stop all clinical and administrative work on May 13, my birthday. I stuck around long enough to follow all my patients after surgery and then retired on August 31, 2013. On my retirement, the entrance foyer of the Mazankowski Alberta Heart Institute was named after me. What an honour. Moreover, the Arvind Koshal Scholarship Fund was created to fund future educational and research endeavours. The good work would go on long after I was gone.

One of the drawbacks of staying in Canada was the distance from my parents. As they grew older, long-haul flights and travel was not feasible for them. My mother always questioned why I could not have worked closer to home. Dubai was often mentioned as an alternative. My father was more practical and knew that the Canadian job was a great opportunity for me. Our visits home were short, dividing our time between Arti's parents and mine. That also left no time for travel in India outside the family homes.

My parents introduced us to Vijay Gupta, a prominent businessman in India. Vijay and his wife Shashi lived in Bhilai, a short distance from Raipur. He had undergone coronary artery bypass surgery in the late 1970s in London and visited us several times in Canada. A great friend, he took care of medical and other issues with our family when we couldn't be there, becoming part of our extended family. I depended on him to keep me informed. Whenever Vijay called about my parents' health and asked me to come over, I knew there was a serious problem and would fly over in haste. My father died in 1999 and Vijay helped me get through those mournful last days. We lost my mother in 2006, and once again, Vijay was on hand to make all the arrangements. I owe him a big debt of gratitude.

Closer to our adopted home in Canada, there was that commanding father figure Dr. Keon. A year after leaving Ottawa, we invited Anne and Wilbert Keon to Edmonton and took them on a trip to the Rocky Mountains, where we all revelled in the breathtaking scenery of Jasper. They both seemed pleased to see how the move had proved right for me.

Dr. Keon remained a senator until he was seventy-five. We continued to support him and stayed connected. He was invited to attend my retirement celebration, where he gave a very thoughtful speech about our times together.

Dr. Keon died at eighty-two years of age in 2019, and I flew from California to attend his funeral in Ottawa. One of his sons, Ryan, told me that his father felt proud of the fact that I had continued his legacy by building the Heart Institute in Edmonton. I was touched. It could never have happened without all I learned from him.

15

Retirement

What does the hard-working cardiac surgeon do in retirement? What fills the days that used to be taken up with one emergency after another? First off: bridge. In retirement, I wanted to get better at the card game. I'd read *Bridge for Dummies*, but with my crazy work schedule I couldn't fit in any face-to-face games so played online. When I came home late in the middle of winter, I'd log on for a game or two. Just to unwind. Playing by the seat of my pants.

I remembered my parents playing bridge—and the vicious arguments they had over games. It was the only time they ever fought. Bidding wars. I'd hear them criticize each other: "Why did you do that?" "What a silly choice that was!" "I never would have come up with that bid." They were just "kitchen bridge" players—which suggests a friendly game around the kitchen table—but those arguments were fierce. It made me think I shouldn't look for games with

Arti, who was an avid player. Perhaps I could find another partner—someone other than my computer.

One day Arti came back from bridge club and said she'd met an older gentleman who asked if she was Dr. Koshal's wife. She'd said yes. "I'd love to see him sometime," he said. "I was one of his patients."

Eighteen years earlier the man had been given only three weeks to live. I operated on him and evidently had saved his life. Alvin Baragar was his name. It was nice to know that he remembered me. Following Arti's lead, we were reintroduced, and he expressed his deep gratitude. Turned out he was a retired professor of math modelling and a champion bridge player. He'd even written some short essays about the game. "Let me play with you," Alvin said.

Me? I barely had 19 master points and Alvin had over 5,000 master points. If we were going to be bridge partners, he couldn't play at a low level like mine. It wasn't permitted. I could play in his tournament league, but he couldn't play in mine. I'd have to play with all the expert players like him. The prospect was terrifying.

"I don't know," I said.

"Let's try it," he said.

And we did. What a great experience that was. I was reminded of something I'd seen and experienced before. When you play—or work—with someone better than you, you learn a lot. You get better. Your game gets better. At least mine did. Everyone around the table was nice to me, and Alvin was a great teacher. Soon we were playing very competitive bridge. I even got confident enough to teach others how to play. From slow learner to teacher.

Arti feels she is better than me, which is a matter of dispute. But that's exactly why we don't play together. Our partnership—so successful in countless ways—would not benefit from such interactions.

THEN THERE WAS golf. I used to play golf and it was on par with what my bridge game used to be. There was a golf course near our house in Edmonton and our kids started playing. Anu was very good. Amit too. Not Arjun: he went for other sports like tennis.

But as the boys got better at golf, we'd go with them to some fabled courses in North America like Pebble Beach, on the Hawaiian islands, and in the Alberta Rocky Mountains where we could enjoy the scenery while watching them play.

If I ever played in Edmonton, I'd often get some emergency phone call in the middle of a game. Whenever I showed up for a game, the inevitable question was: "So, Dr. Koshal, how many holes will you be playing today?" Good question, since the customary nine or eighteen wasn't a given. Once when I was on the course I had to speak to the minister of health, which I did—in the middle of the fairway, thanks to the mobility of cellphone communication.

The season for golf was rather short up in our part of Canada. Not a lot of time to practice. But then in retirement, we ended up buying a home in the California desert—I'll get to that—and from November through April, there was one good day after another to play. My game improved. In fact, my experience as a heart surgeon helped. I was used to having to learn new things and work under enormous pressure. Standing there at the tee ready to swing my club,

I'd remind myself, "It's just a game." Not quite like standing in the OR with my gloves on, ready to operate, but calming nonetheless.

Not long ago I actually won a tournament at our course in Indian Wells. There were a lot of people standing around watching, checking us out. It made some of my friends a little nervous. Not me. I was used to the attention. I could be calm and cool. After all, hadn't I performed heart transplants for an audience? This was my retirement crowd.

I PROMISED ARTI I wouldn't be a burden to her in this phase of life. "You're never going to have to make breakfast or lunch for me ever again," I said. I would do it.

Talk about a steep learning curve. I had never cooked. I could barely boil an egg. As a kid I wasn't even allowed in the kitchen. But I was determined to change that. I wanted to make some of those good vegetarian Indian dishes for lunch, favourite things like puri, a deep-fried crispy yet soft Indian bread. (Arti will challenge me by saying it's not heart healthy, which it isn't, but if you don't eat it all the time...) It's especially tasty with curried potatoes and yogurt. What a heavenly smell. "If you can do heart surgery," I told myself, "you should be able to make a dish." It's not like I wasn't used to holding a knife.

I got on the Internet, downloaded recipes, clicked onto YouTube and watched some master chefs at work. Good teachers all. Doing what they said, I got better and better. I also found that cooking—seeing and touching and smelling the ingredients that went into a dish—made me more appreciative of what I ate, whether it was from Arti's hand or at some nice restaurant. Cooking always had some mystique for me, but it wasn't all that hard. And Arti's compliments meant worlds to me.

Now for breakfast I'd do some fried eggs with hash browns, maybe oatmeal too, or I'd cook up a batch of French toast for the family if the boys and their families were visiting. Lunch could be quesadillas, pizza, salads, fish and chips. Delicious. Sometimes I'll cook up fried dahivada, made with lentils in yogurt. It costs only $5 to make, but I'd choose it over a $50 piece of sea bass. Reminds me of what we ate at Montessori school all those years ago. And my big hit is salmon on rice topped with layers of mint, mango, and cilantro and served with ketjap manis sauce. It's not the results that matter but the pleasure of losing myself in the work, cooking, cleaning up ... I'm now a regular at emptying the dishwasher, knowing exactly where everything should go. At least I think so.

Add to that, puttering around the house, fixing things like the flapper valve on the toilet, or screwing in a new light bulb. (No Alex next door to tease me.) There was a scratch on the golf cart, and I enjoyed the challenge of finding just the right colour of paint and touching it up.

Here's the truth of the matter: I've never been bored in retirement. Not for a moment. I don't read as much as I used to. Occasionally I take in an article or two in a medical journal, seeing how my profession keeps growing and changing, but there's always something to do. Watch some cricket on TV, like I did as a kid. Go out to dinner with friends. Play pickleball. And bridge and golf.

WE KNEW THAT the harsh Edmonton winters wouldn't be conducive to our lifestyle. After all, we didn't grow up with snow and ice and didn't ski or skate. From time to time, we would take short breaks to go south, vacation trips to California, Arizona, Nevada. A lot of my patients talked about their favourite warm spots for the winter and how they either rented or owned homes.

At the same time, Arti always talked about how she wanted to travel around the world. I couldn't afford to take long vacations while I was working. I promised her that I would take her wherever she wanted to go when I retired. Indeed, we've now been to Spain, Italy, London, Hong Kong, South Africa, Vietnam, and Cambodia; we've taken a cruise on the Rhine and a trip through the Mekong River Delta. And the list of destinations keeps growing. Go see the Grand Canyon, go for a safari in Tanzania, visit the island of Java.

In hindsight, I should have put an end date to my promise!

In February 2013, a few months before I retired, we made an important decision. Palm Springs was an easy direct flight from Edmonton. That's where we'd buy our winter house. Arti took the lead in finding just the right place. After sorting through a host of different communities and resorts, she selected a house in the Reserve Golf Club in Indian Wells that came well recommended by our real estate agent and some friends. We consulted our kids. Amit said we should not wait; at the time, the Canadian dollar and US dollar were at par and the prices were reasonable. We've never looked back.

I've often wished my parents were still alive and could come visit. They'd love it. The balmy weather, the warm sunshine, the friendly community, the good food—we probably eat out more nights than we cook at home—bridge games that don't end up in arguments. I remember getting word back in 1999 that my father was failing fast. I flew to India and was there for the end. His last words to me were, "Namaste." His farewell, his greeting. When I flew over to see my mother in her last days in 2006, I got word shortly after landing, before I could reach her bedside, that she had died just then. Her last words were, "Arvind's landed." Somehow, she knew.

What also struck me hard was the loss of my beloved sister Reeni, only thirteen months older than I am. She fell, broke her hip, had surgery, got an infection, and went downhill fast. I longed to be there by her side, but in those early days of the COVID pandemic, I couldn't travel to India. No one could. I mourned the loss from afar. Arti's mother is still alive, and Arti goes back to see her regularly; with my life remade on this side of the Atlantic, my visits to India will continue but not as often.

What has certainly made a difference is watching our three sons grow and thrive. Arjun is a lawyer in New York, currently COO of the non-profit New York Structural Biology Center after eighteen years with Simpson Thacher, a prestigious New York law firm. Anu first got a PhD from Duke in comparative litera-ture and philosophy, then went to Toronto for his law degree, and is now a partner at McCarthy Tétrault, a prestigious law firm in Canada, and is a tax litigator. And Amit, after getting a PhD in finance from MIT, is the money manager for a large family port-folio based in Edmonton. They're all happily married, and we have three wonderful daughters-in-law, not to mention five adorable grandchildren.

I might be retired—happily—but the inner cardiac surgeon is still at work. Out in California where our community of houses wrap around a golf course, I learned of a man who was struck by a heart attack in Long Beach, not far away. He was on a golf course there and the only reason he survived is that he was on the 18th hole, not far from the pro shop, close to a defibrillator and help.

What if there was some emergency like that on our golf course? How long would it take an ambulance to get there? The course wasn't especially close to the road—that was part of its appeal. And the only way to reach most parts of it was by golf cart. What if we equipped a golf cart with the necessary items to help someone in a heart emergency? What if we had a defibrillator right there, and a gurney where a patient could lie, and a wooden plank to put underneath if needed for CPR?

I spoke to my friends on the board of our club and the idea appealed to them. We'd get a golf cart for this very purpose. I had to stress that it wouldn't be a golf cart ambulance per se. It wouldn't have everything an ambulance had (no EMTs!), but it would be capable of transporting someone who was sick or injured and reaching anyone who needed help on the course. We'd also need to train the staff in how to do CPR and use a defibrillator—like a fire extinguisher in your home, it won't do a lot of good if you don't know how to use it. We'd also have to make sure that training was regularly updated for existing staff and included for new employees coming on board.

Emergency preparedness can become lax when there are no emergencies to respond to.

That emergency golf cart was on hand, parked near the clubhouse, for several years before it was pressed into service. I was playing golf with a friend and at the 3rd hole he started getting wobbly and immediately sat in a golf cart. I checked his pulse: 120. I asked him if he'd had anything to drink. No—so I gave him some water. He insisted he wanted to keep playing. He seemed to be okay, so we kept playing—he was actually playing quite well. But then on the 16th hole, I found him unable to walk up out of a sand bunker. We helped him to his golf cart. His pulse had plummeted to 40. We dialed 911 and called for the golf cart medical transport. It was there in eight minutes. We put him on the gurney, lifted his legs, and got him stabilized. I could keep an eye on his pulse until an ambulance arrived twenty minutes later. They took him to the hospital, and he survived.

I'm glad I was there, glad I could help, but someday I won't be. Yet the means of survival will be on hand with people trained to help. We now have a similar medical cart at the Royal Mayfair Golf Club in Edmonton. A well-equipped emergency golf cart as my legacy? It's easier to point to all the patients whose lives I played a role in saving, like my bridge partner. Not the fruits of my labour alone, just the actions I was able to take with all the people on hand who helped. Don't put my name on that special golf cart, but I am secretly—okay, maybe not so secretly—proud of it. What a way to keep living the life I was called to.

Cardiac surgeon. It wasn't what I planned. It wasn't even in my parents' vision. But it happened and how glad I am that it did. People are talking about how the profession is changing, like the advent of stents and devices like the TAVR (transcatheter aortic valve replacement) that don't require open-heart surgery to be implanted and that make for an easier recovery. I'm a doctor. Patients come first. Whatever is best for them. What an amazing era we live in when what can be done for heart patients has expanded by leaps and bounds.

How fortunate I was to be a part of it. Take it from this grateful cardiac surgeon.

Looking Back

n 1982, seven years after I left India, my wonderful teacher and mentor there, Dr. Atm Prakash, had a massive heart attack and died at the All India Institute of Medical Sciences in New Delhi where I had trained. As was then the practice, he was treated medically, not surgically. An intelligent man and himself a surgeon, he was not convinced of the cardiac surgical expertise offered in India. I was shocked and saddened, especially for his children and young wife. I felt his loss personally, especially since he was instrumental in my coming to Canada. I wished he had opted for an angiogram and, if needed, coronary artery surgery, which would have been life-saving. But I understood the context of his decision: the systemic challenges and shortcomings that existed within the health care landscape in India. And which I had come to see in Canada as well. Those realizations fuelled my determination to effect positive change from within the system, and had a profound impact on how I thought about serving patients—as a doctor, an administrator, and a lifelong learner. I became acutely aware that improvements were within our reach, offering the opportunity to save more lives.

Later on, in my Edmonton practice, I remember a patient coming to my office ten years after he had had coronary artery bypass. He was looking somewhat downcast. "What is the matter?" I asked. "Aren't I going to die now?" he asked. "No, no," I insisted. At the time of his surgery, there was a belief that his particular operation only lasted for ten years because the vein grafts commonly used tended to close over time. In his case, for the graft we had used a mammary artery (from behind his sternum). With the introduction of new techniques and technologies, a small artery such as the mammary could be successfully used as a bypass, resulting in patients leading much longer lives. My patient is still in good health and recently turned ninety— the kind of success story that is one of the rewards of my profession.

When we speak of innovation in medicine, our minds tend to gravitate toward technological advancements and novel techniques, many of which have been a part of my cardiac surgery practice and which I have described in this book. Undoubtedly, these advancements have saved countless lives. However, innovation is not confined to technological marvels. It encompasses the constant pursuit of improving and transforming care through people and processes. These, too, I've been privileged to experience, and to be a part of, in my career.

In the latter context, I reflect upon the collective efforts of my fellow physicians, nurses, administrators, officials, researchers, technicians, support staff, and countless others across the nation. Their profound dedication has propelled an incremental but remarkable shift in the landscape of cardiovascular care, toppling heart disease from its perch as the leading cause of death in Canada. This is an embodiment of a health care system whose fundamental mission is to provide equitable care to all its citizens. It is a tale of working collectively within that system to continually enhance its efficacy and impact.

WHAT I'VE RECOUNTED in this book is not precisely what my father envisaged when he chose this profession for me in India, nor is it what Arti foresaw when she became my life partner. Even Dr. Prakash could not have foreseen that I would stay in Canada, where he too had trained, and contribute in the way I have. That said, it is a story of immense pride and accomplishment—a testament to unwavering dedication and collaborative spirit in the pursuit of patient well-being—my story, yes, but also a quintessentially Canadian story.

Afterword

My three sons have always been helpful when I ask for advice, even in administrative matters. It has been interesting to gain their perspective on the issues I faced at work, which provided me with valuable insights into that environment. After retiring, I had the opportunity to give a talk about my experiences at work at the Reserve Club in Indian Wells, California, which was well received. Amit was in the audience and turned to Arti, saying, "I had no idea Dad went through all of this." Arti then suggested that I document my working life, and thus began the journey of writing this book.

Over a two-year period, I wrote the first several pages. Encouraged by this progress, I sought the expertise of an experienced author. Enter Rick Hamlin. He had published several of his own books and had helped others in similar situations. Rick and I worked closely together to bring this book to its current form. Working with him was a pleasure, as he skillfully translated my words, memories, thoughts, and feelings onto the page. His contribution was invaluable.

Arjun also collaborated with Rick and me, playing an instrumental role in encouraging me to expand the book beyond its original draft and helped refine the manuscript for publication. Arjun's wife, Melissa Jun Koshal, a graphic designer in New York, helped with the original draft and designed the book cover. Once again, this endeavour was a team effort.

As I continue moving forward in life, I derive immense joy from witnessing the accomplishments of my sons and their families, as they raise their own children and excel in their chosen professions. Observing what I missed but didn't realize I was missing is truly fulfilling. They are dedicated, hands-on parents who relish being an active part of their children's lives—a role that I was unable to fully fulfill. Coming from a generation that believed my duty as a husband and father was to provide for my family by working hard and doing my best, I feel content knowing I gave it my all, and that my wife and children know and understand that.

I hope that one day my five grandchildren will comprehend the efforts their grandpa undertook to make their parents' lives the best they could be.

The Questions I'm Most Often Asked About Heart Surgery

What is the best place to choose for surgery?

With all the time and effort we spent developing the Mazankow-ski Alberta Heart Institute in Edmonton, you shouldn't be surprised that I've put this question first. Place matters. There might be more than one heart centre in your area. Check them all out. In some big cities, there may be dozens within easy driving distance. In other regions, there may be only one or two. You want the best in the area.

A lot depends on how unusual your issue is. Some operations are so simple they can be done anywhere. Others demand extensive experience. If your condition is complex, it is worthwhile to go further afield. It's a little like getting your car repaired. Can you go to the guy around the corner, or do you need a special appointment with the dealership? It all depends. Same with you and your heart.

Some things to consider: Does the place have a dedicated cardiac ICU or would heart patients be included as part of the general ICU?

Is it well equipped to handle any complications that might come up? Can it put you on an assist device if there's any sort of problem? If this is a second time for open-heart surgery, you want to be especially cautious. Cutting through the sternum takes less than a minute if it's the first time. It's far more complicated the second time around.

The smaller hospitals can do simpler operations, such as:

- first-time coronary bypass surgery
- first-time heart valve repair/replacement
- other simpler operations such as getting a pacemaker, defibrillator, or coronary stent (usually done by a cardiologist)

Complex cases should be done in a bigger centre. These include second- or third-time open-heart surgery, or combined procedures such as coronary bypass and valve surgery, as well as surgery for an aortic aneurysm.

What are the risks of the operation?

You need to talk to the surgeon and ask some difficult questions. Bring a loved one with you to help you ask the questions and *hear* the answers. Neither is easy at such a stressful time. You need to be blunt though. Find out: What is the risk of dying? What is the risk of getting a stroke or an infection? Be specific. Your surgeon needs to tell you. Also ask: What are the risks of dying with versus without the operation? What is the risk if surgery is postponed? For how long could it be postponed? Ask about the surgeon's practice:

How many such operations has the surgeon done and/or do they do, say, monthly? What is their success rate for the procedure? How experienced is the surgeon, and is the quality of experience germane to your particular situation?

Let's say there's a one or two per cent chance of you dying. Of course, that's small, but it's very good to know. You'll want to make sure your affairs are in order. Are there any financial matters you need to settle? Do you have a will? Use this as a moment to update any plans. Don't take things for granted. Once again, a family member, a loved one, a close friend can be your advocate and ally. You'll have enough to worry about as you recover from surgery. You don't want any unfinished business hanging over your head. Or heart.

Google the heart surgeon. Google the centre where the surgeon works. Google the patient reviews. Most likely your cardiologist has referred you to the surgeon. If so, ask for more than one name. Also ask your cardiologist—frankly—what their experience is with those surgeons. What do they know of them? How many of their patients have gone to one versus the other? And of course, be wary of any sales pitches. Like buying a new car, you don't decide based on what the ads say. Do a little more research of your own. Or again, ask for a loved one's help.

If your surgeon can do the operation immediately—and it's not an emergency—be a bit suspicious. The best surgeons have a waiting list. They are in high demand. Check with the secretary. For open-heart surgeries, you want someone who has done the procedure at least a few hundred times. For less invasive surgeries, again volume of surgeries is important. Is it a repair job or a replacement? If it's a mitral valve, it should be repaired whenever possible. It should be replaced only if a repair is not feasible. On the other hand, an aortic valve should be replaced, and only occasionally repaired depending on the surgeon's experience. If it's a minimally invasive approach, ensure that the surgeon has done a sufficient number. Find out where the surgeon learned these procedures. Be careful if they're suggesting robotic surgery. It has not been a big success in cardiac surgery.

A TAVR (trans catheter aortic valve replacement) is less invasive and might be a good choice, but don't go for it for that reason alone. The procedure is suitable for patients who are at risk for open-heart surgery, but the traditional approach still remains the best.

Can a larger artificial valve be used to replace a damaged valve?

In open-heart surgery to replace your aortic valve, the old diseased valve is taken out and a new larger valve is put in its place. This is different from TAVR, where the old valve can't be removed, so a new valve is put inside it. The size of the new valve matters a lot for how well you'll do after the surgery. Artificial heart valves have been developed over the years. The two main choices are tissue—made out of animal tissues and occasionally a human preserved homograft—or mechanical—made of pyrolytic carbon. The current tissue valves and the mechanical valves are longer-lasting, but the downside to the mechanical valve is that the patient will need to be on blood thinners like Warfarin (Coumadin) for the rest of their days. If you're an athlete, that can be a real burden. And a possible danger. In conversation with your surgeon and cardiologist those issues must be addressed.

What will recovery be like?

An aortic valve replacement will require from four to ten days of recovery in the hospital. A TAVR replacement may only require two or three days. This is why a dedicated heart centre is especially valuable. After surgery, there is an ICU right there for the patient's initial recovery, with experienced nurses and doctors around to monitor every aspect of that recovery.

At the Heart Institute we made a point of moving patients out of the ICU and into a room as soon as possible, using in-house physiotherapy and rehabilitation. In general, when you're able to walk up two flights of stairs, you're ready to go home. And then at home, being an outpatient with follow-up visits from a nurse. It wasn't just to free up beds but also for the patient's recovery. Being at home and rebuilding strength in a familiar environment. And then when they're ready to return for cardiac rehab, generally a month or two after surgery. Step by step you resume regular life—possibly even doing it better. Having guidance in getting back to regular cardiovascular exercise and having a heart-healthy diet.

Access to tele health for patients living far from the main hospital is a useful tool for follow-up care without making long trips.

Endnotes

1. E.S. Nicholls, J. Jung, and J.W. Davies, "Cardiovascular Disease Mortality in Canada," *CMA Journal 125* (November 1, 1981): 981–992. www.ncbi.nlm.nih.gov/pmc/articles/PMC1862487 /pdf/canmedaj01354-0039.pdf.

2. THE DAILY – Deaths, 2021, "Cancer and Heart Disease Remain the Two Top Leading Causes of Death in Canada." www150.statcan.gc.ca/n1/daily-quotidien/230828/dq230828b -eng.htm#.

3. Ian Aird, *A Companion in Surgical Studies* (Edinburgh: E. & S. Livingstone, Ltd., 1949).

4. A. Koshal, M.M. Krausz, et al. "Preservation of Platelets and Their Function in Prolonged CPB Using Prostacyclin," *Circulation* 64 (2 Pt 2) (Aug 1981): II44–48.

5. A. Koshal, D.S. Beanlands, et al. "Urgent Surgical Reperfusion in Acute Evolving Myocardial Infarction: A Randomized Controlled Study," *Circulation* 78 (3 Pt 2) (Sep 1988): II71–78.

6. Lisa Priest and Katherine Harding, "Baby Xander's Life-saving Transplant," *Globe and Mail*, February 18, 2006, front page.

7. L. Elder, "History of Jehovah's Witnesses," National Institutes of Health, 2008. www.ncbi.nlm.nih.gov › articles › PMC2529448.

Index

Pattison, Jim, 170
pediatric cardiac surgery
    challenges of confidence in
        programs for, 137
    challenges of out-of-province
        procedures, 136–37
    high mortality rate in, 137
    improvement to University of
        Alberta Hospitals' program
        for, 139–43
    lack of in 1991, 133
Peter Bent Brigham Hospital
    (Boston), 63
Pipe, Andrew, 47, 90, 92, 95,
    100
Prakash, Atm, 27, 28, 29, 37, 38,
    195

R
Ravishankar University Medical
    College, 18–19
Rebeyka, Ivan, 140–42, 166
Regional Cardiac Sciences
    program, 176, 180
residents
    and accreditation reviews, 128
    AK's mentorship of, 129
    AK's vision of program for,
        125, 126–27
    demands on, 124
    importance of, 123, 131,
        132–33
    undervaluing of, 124–25
    See also surgical training
    process

Robinson, Reverend Canon J.E.,
    13, 83
Ross, David, 141–42
Rotary Club, 81
Royal Alexandra Hospital
    (Edmonton), 151, 180
Royal College of Physicians and
    Surgeons (Canada), 51, 66,
    128, 129–31
Royal College of Surgeons
    (UK), 4, 5
Royal Mayfair Golf Club
    (Edmonton), 193
Royal Postgraduate Medical
    School (UK), 4

S
Safdarjung Hospital
    (New Delhi), 27
Scindia School, 10
Shaw, John Robert ("JR"), 165,
    166
Shaw Cablesystems, 165
Sheila bai, 10
SickKids. *See* Hospital for Sick
    Children
Singh, Arjun (Mr. and Mrs.),
    32, 37
Singh, Veena, 32, 33, 37
Sondhi family, 2
Southey, Robert, 13, 83
St. Boniface Hospital
    (Winnipeg), 146, 148
St. Joseph's Convent School, 12
St. Michael's Hospital
    (Toronto), 90